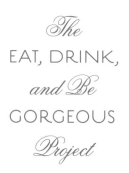

The
EAT, DRINK,
and Be
GORGEOUS
Project

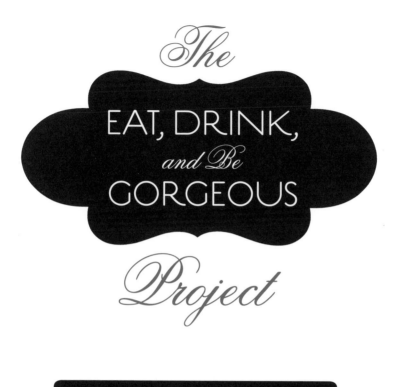

The

EAT, DRINK, and Be GORGEOUS

Project

THREE MONTHS TO A NEW YOU

ESTHER BLUM, M.S., R.D., C.D.N., C.N.S.,
AUTHOR OF *EAT, DRINK, AND BE GORGEOUS*

CHRONICLE BOOKS
SAN FRANCISCO

ISBN: 978-1-4521-0258-0

Manufactured in China

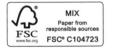

Designed by Andrew Schapiro

10 9 8 7 6 5 4 3 2 1

Chronicle Books LLC
680 Second Street
San Francisco, California 94107
www.chroniclebooks.com

FOR ROBERT CRAYHON
friend, mentor, comedian, and healer.

I OWE THIS ALL TO YOU.

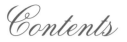

Contents

INTRODUCTION

Who doesn't love a good project, especially when that project is *you*? After all, there isn't a woman out there who doesn't want to do better for herself. Bearing in mind that love of self is the best love, I'm putting this project out into the world to help you change the way you think and to give you loads of techniques to help you do better. It will turn your "won't power" into willpower. You will learn tools and tricks from some of the best experts in the field. And, although it may not be easy at first, in time you'll learn to be the mistress of your own domain. And that's what being gorgeous is all about—being empowered, armed, and dangerously curved.

Keeping track of what you eat is one of the best forms of cognitive behavioral therapy. Not only does it rewire your brain and incite change, but it also brings awareness and focus to what you put in your mouth. If you bite it, you write it! A food diary is the highest form of personal accountability and will quickly help you identify imbalances in your ratios of proteins, carbohydrates, and fat.

The mission of this project is to help you create awareness (and change, if necessary) of what you are eating and draw conclusions from that information—just as a personalized counseling session would. Did you gain more energy from changing the way you eat? Lose weight? Stop eating that daily extra piece of chocolate? Go for a walk on the weekend instead of lying on the couch? It's all about inspiring you to eat healthfully and create motivation and change within yourself.

The Eat, Drink, and Be Gorgeous Project contains cutting-edge information on exercise, supplements, and clean eating. You'll learn how to make your food work for you—not the other way around. Check out the "Gorgeously Fit" chapter to learn how to maximize your fat-burning potential. At the end of this book are four different meal plan options to choose from. Go with the one that fits your goals and give it a whirl for a month—I promise you'll have a different body in four weeks. You can stay on any of these plans as long as you like, or toggle back and forth between them as your needs change. I've also included recipes for starters, mains, sides, and desserts to bust up boredom in the kitchen. They may even expand your recipe repertoire so much that you're inspired to throw that fabulous dinner party you've been thinking about. You'll find question-and-answer sections at the end of each chapter that should satisfy your own questions and help you realize that your challenges are not solely your own; everyone needs support when making changes. And, of course, you'll have three months' worth of food diary pages. Yep, I'm here with you for the long haul!

You may think that just because I write these books this is all a snap for me. Think again! Being a registered dietitian does not necessarily make it easy for me to eat healthfully all the time; I struggle to consistently eat well just like you do! After all, I'm still a human with cravings, weaknesses, and a lot of other priorities to manage beyond what I put in my body. Eating mindfully takes time, practice, and commitment. And doing the very best you can every day is all you can ask of yourself. I know from years of having counseled thousands of women that if you try your best every day *and* keep a food and exercise log, you'll start to see real results.

Planning for a couple of weekly splurges can also help keep you honest the rest of the time. When my own motivation slips, I often look to my like-minded fitness and foodie friends for inspiration. You know the people I mean—the ones who really walk the walk and keep it real with consistent workouts and by eating right. After all, who among us would truly be successful without a partner or mentor in reaching our goals?

You may have had a specific goal in mind when you picked up *The Eat, Drink, and Be Gorgeous Project.* Perhaps you want to lose weight, change your body, eat better, or embrace healthier lifestyle habits. Perhaps you just need a support system. But no matter what, you want to love life while achieving your goals, right? Whatever your final destination, you've come to the right place. This is a judgment-free zone, where you can learn personal accountability and learn about what motivates you to stay on track. You may also figure out what road blocks are standing in your way, enabling you to break through and let go of behaviors that are no longer working for you. Just remember that your process of building behavioral changes is even more important than your goal of getting fit, because your process is what will enable you to make lifelong changes. Find your goal, commit to your vision, and realize your dream!

Stay Gorgeous!

Esther

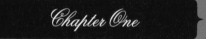

Chapter One

EATING GORGEOUSLY

The best (and really, the only) way to change your lifestyle and way of eating is to commit to get fit and be consistent about it. This means planning your meals in advance and spending sufficient time grocery shopping, either in person or online, and cooking each week. If you don't have much time to cook during the week, choose a weekend day to do prep work: washing and storing produce, and cooking and freezing soups, stews, meatballs, burgers, brown rice, beans, and sweet potatoes. You will also need to invest in safe, nonplastic reusable containers to make your food and drinks portable. This preparation effort is at the heart of your success and may very possibly test your level of commitment. Know that you are not alone; this is a challenge for my clients and myself as well. So here's the takeaway: If you fail to plan, you plan to fail. But if you plan ahead, then the world is your oyster—and quite a delicious one at that!

The Real Deal

"If it doesn't run, fly, swim, or grow from the ground, it's not food!"

I come back to this quote by Annemarie Colbin again and again. When reading labels, you can try following this rule of thumb: If you can't ID it, don't eat it! The fewer ingredients a product has, the less guesswork you need to do to determine if a food is right for you. Stick to the basics, and keep it simple with whole foods. Proteins, fruits, vegetables, legumes, brown rice, nuts, and seeds will give your body the building blocks it needs to help you feel energized, build lean muscle, burn fat, and let go of toxins and unwanted weight. Live gorgeously; eat mindfully.

Rx for Weight Loss

One important point I'd like you to take away from this book is this: For making long-term changes in your physique, the low-calorie model for weight loss is obsolete. On the contrary, high-protein foods take more work to digest, metabolize, and use, which means you burn more calories processing them. And eating adequate protein ensures that you keep your precious muscle tissue—something that is often lost with a low-calorie diet. In a study published in *Nutrition Metabolism*, dieters who increased their protein intake to 30 percent of their diet ate nearly 450 fewer calories a day and lost about 11 lb/5 kg during 12 weeks without employing any other dietary measures. Here's the key, though: Your best flat-belly bets are found in complete proteins like skinless chicken or turkey, eggs and egg whites, seafood, pork, venison, buffalo, ostrich, and lean beef (ideally grass fed). Vegetarians will need to be a little more creative and nosh on fermented soy like tempeh, *natto*, and miso; hemp seed and hemp protein powder; pea protein powder; rice protein powder; buckwheat; and quinoa. Complementary proteins like beans and rice, natural peanut butter on hemp bread, and brown rice with chopped pecans are a must as well.

Protein Prowess

In order to create change within your body, you must change the way you eat; exercise alone will not reduce your body fat or build lean muscle unless you give it the tools it needs. Women need far more protein than you might think. I would never have believed it myself, until I befriended a group of female bodybuilding competitors. How much protein is enough for us ladies? A good range to shoot for is roughly 1 g of protein per 1 lb/0.5 kg of body weight. So a 140-lb/63-kg woman would need to consume 18 to 22 oz/455 to 625 g of protein per day, or roughly 5 oz/140 g per meal plus another 2 oz/55 g at each snack. It's also critical to get at least 5 oz/140 g of that protein at breakfast (this would equal two whole eggs plus two whites or one to two scoops of whey protein powder mixed into a smoothie) to replenish your protein stores after fasting all night and keep your appetite in check throughout the day. Keep your protein intake pretty consistent, even on the days you're not working out, because you are building and repairing the most muscle tissue on those precious rest days while helping your body lose fat. It may sound shocking, but it actually makes a whole lot of sense when you think about the anabolic effects that protein has upon lean muscle tissue. So if you've been exercising for years and haven't seen the changes you'd like in your body, now is the time to incorporate new habits into your regime. The secret to a rock-hard body isn't eating according to the traditional Food Guide Pyramid or the more recent My Plate recommendations; it's eating large amounts of high-quality proteins throughout the day, limited amounts of complex carbo-hydrates and fats, and lifting heavy weights three to four times per week. Throw in 30 minutes of high-intensity interval training three times per week and you're on your way to being in the best shape of your life.

The Carb Window

Milton Berle said, "If opportunity doesn't knock, build a door." I say, if you want to eat carbs, open a window! The best time for you to eat your favorite sweet carbs (think bananas, figs, pineapple, or even a couple of squares of dark chocolate) is within 30 minutes of finishing your workout. Eating sugary carbs immediately following a workout will spike your insulin levels, and during this window this metabolic surge can help you build muscle tissue. The same goes for coffee, which also spikes insulin and cortisol; it should be consumed 30 minutes before or after your workouts. Otherwise, it will just raise cortisol levels, but without glucagon present to counteract the effects.

Morning, Sunshine!

What's the best bevvie to start your day off right? Hot cocoa! Drinking 1 tbsp of unrefined, organic cocoa powder in 8 oz/240 ml of hot water will give your brain the happy neurotransmitter, serotonin, while giving your adrenals a shot of energy. Cocoa helps reduce cravings, is high in antioxidants, and won't make you jittery and irritable. If you really can't quit the java, then mix 1 tbsp cocoa powder and a dash of cinnamon in your coffee to blunt the stress-inducing and weight-gaining effects of cortisol. The organic acids in both decaf and regular coffee can raise cortisol levels and accelerate the aging process, so go for the gold with cocoa instead! Try it hot in the winter and iced in the summer; sweeten with xylitol or stevia powder for a rich, guilt-free treat. I love to dump 1 tbsp cocoa powder into a protein smoothie; it tastes like you're drinking a Fudgesicle!

Gluten-Free and Gorgeous!

Want to drop 6 to 10 percent of your body fat in one month? Then go gluten-free. No matter where you are on the gluten sensitivity spectrum, almost everyone feels better off the wacky junk. Think about it this way: Gluten is present in all processed foods. Most of us eat at least one gluten-containing processed food on a daily basis (a slice of bread, cereal, crackers, and so on). So just by eliminating packaged foods, you're clearing out metabolic roadblocks from your diet, because even the slightest sensitivity to a food can cause you to retain water and prevent you from losing body fat. More important, clearing out gluten-containing carbs forces you to eat more whole foods like lentils, winter squash, sweet potatoes, proteins, nuts and avocadoes, and fresh fruits and vegetables. Now, if you'll excuse me, I'm off to enjoy my steak salad with a side of butternut squash soup!

Bloat Busters

If you compete with camels when it comes to water retention, try incorporating these bloat busters into your daily diet: asparagus, celery, cranberries, and 2 tbsp of unsweetened cranberry juice in water. All of these foods help the body release extra stored fluid, which can make you appear as if you weigh more than you actually do. Replace your salt with fresh herbs and salt-free seasonings, horse-radish, wasabi, mustard, cayenne, and Tabasco sauce. Don't forget to pop a supplement with 50 mg of B_6 and 1,000 mg of taurine to help the body gently release extra water. Also be mindful of alcohol intake; even one drink can cause you to retain 3 to 4 lb/1.4 to 1.8 kg of water for up to five days afterward!

Show Your True Colors

Putting colors on your plate is top notch when it comes to longevity. *Orange* foods benefit the eyes and skin: mangoes, sweet potatoes, winter squash, pumpkin, cantaloupe, apricots, and carrots. Lycopene is present in *red* foods and reduces the risk of cancer: tomatoes, watermelon, guava, and pink grapefruit. Anthocyanins are found in *red* and *purple* foods: cabbage, red and purple grapes, red wine, cherries, blueberries, acai berries, strawberries, blackberries, cranberries, eggplant, plums, prunes, red pear, and red peppers. These foods protect your heart, brain, and eyes. Don't forget the garden-variety *green* foods like kale, broccoli, Brussels sprouts, and spinach, which will detoxify your liver and alka-linize your rockin' bod, and *yellow* foods like yellow peppers, summer squash, lemons, and bananas, which are also rich in phytonutrients. Plants do a body good!

On the Go?

With our eat-on-the-run culture, we don't always have the option to eat perfectly all the time. Think "good-better-best" and make the best choices with the options you have. The best thing you can do is plan ahead and always carry one or two snacks with you so you can keep your eye on the prize. While protein is good for you, making it portable can be challenging for some people. After all, not everyone wants to carry a grilled chicken breast around in their bag! If this is the case, try these other portable options: raw nuts, fresh fruit, protein bars (try Power Crunch, Standard Process, or Biogenesis), beef or bison jerky, cut-up fresh veggies, and hard-boiled eggs are all gluten- and dairy-free options that won't clutter up your metabolism and will help keep you right on track. Certainly, if you have access to a fridge or kitchen during the day, then feel free to store roasted chicken, turkey, cans of low-mercury tuna and wild Alaskan salmon, and raw nuts in there to give yourself the cleanest proteins available. Some of my clients who work in sales and are frequently out in the field keep a cooler with snacks in the car to help them adhere to their plan. It's amazing what you can accomplish when you set your mind to it!

Dining Divinely

Dining out can throw even the most well-intended babes off track. Supersize portions, unknown ingredients, and the dreaded bread basket can divert our attention away from the task of clean eating. Not to worry, your Cherry Godmother is here with some savvy tricks of the trade! Follow my rules and you'll be able to look yourself in the mirror tomorrow morning without an iota of regret:

- Before heading out on the town, peruse local restaurant menus online to find one that's in sync with your goals. A steakhouse is great if you're eating for a lean body, whereas a sushi bar will have plenty of gluten-free options.
- At the table, preemptively send the bread basket back. Nobody has that much willpower.
- Double up on vegetables and ditch the starch. This applies especially if you're having a glass of wine.
- Eat your protein first at meals, then your vegetables, then the starch. Have soup or a salad for an appetizer so you fill up on the good stuff first. Protein signals the hypothalamus to turn off hunger signals in the brain, so you fill up more quickly if you eat your protein first.

- When you order salads, request your dressing on the side for some drench control. Dip your fork in the dressing, and then punch it into the lettuce. This trick will save you more calories than you'd think. Keep it pure and simple with olive oil and balsamic vinegar or fresh lemon.
- Practice putting your fork down between bites and don't just shove it all down your gullet. Smells, textures, and flavors will enhance your sensual experience of eating. Take your time! This will help you feel fuller, too.
- If you're full before you're done eating, immediately have the rest of your meal wrapped up. For me, leftovers are the best part of eating out, because they mean one more meal I won't have to cook!
- If you've been eating in a healthy way and working out for at least five consecutive days, then splurge on a reward meal. This means your favorite entrée plus a glass of wine and dessert. Then get back in the saddle at your next meal—no exceptions, cowgirl.

Letting Go of the Weight

It always fascinates me to watch what folks buy at the grocery store. Try to be mindful of the long-term outcomes of a cart full of chocolate bars, ginger snaps, and chocolate-covered raisins—they don't always do a body good! Often the largest roadblock to change is shortsightedness. One cookie per day won't kill you, but it won't enable your body to burn fat, either. Keep yourself on track by writing down what you eat and scheduling weekly indulgences; keep it clean and tight the rest of the time. The farther off track you go, the farther you will have to come back, so be good to yourself and commit to get fit. As my favorite skinny dude, Gandhi, said, "Strength does not come from physical capacity. It comes from an indomitable will."

Out with Flabulous, In with Fabulous!

Get your six-pack abs started in your kitchen with some delicious replacements for old, tired, unhealthy habits. Literally lighten your load by incorporating some incredibly healthful options into your eating plans!

INSTEAD OF . . .	TRY . . .
Potato chips	Turkey jerky
Spaghetti	High-fiber pasta, 100% buckwheat noodles, or spaghetti squash served with meat sauce
Slice of bread	Hemp bread or baked sweet potato
Hamburger and fries	Buffalo burger, no bun, baked sweet potato fries
Ketchup	Salsa
Milk	Almond milk
Gatorade	Coconut water
Cream	Coconut milk creamer
Red Bull	Fresh-brewed iced tea
Soda	Seltzer with a splash of POM pomegranate juice
Salt	Sea salt and/or fresh herbs and spices
Sugar	Stevia, xylitol, erythritol, raw honey, or maple syrup
Beer	Vodka on the rocks, or with club soda on ice
Pizza	Salad with chicken, fresh mozzarella, and tomatoes
Ice cream	So Delicious coconut milk frozen dessert (dairy free)

Keep a list of all the changes you make as each week goes by. Aim for two changes per month to keep your goals simple and realistic. By the end of three months you should notice a big difference in the way you look and feel.

Paleocarbs versus Neocarbs

What the hell are paleocarbs and neocarbs? The answer lies within our agricultural timeline of grain production—and it also addresses a piece of our growing global obesity crisis. Paleocarbs are composed of the carbs that sustained hunter-gatherers; they are nutrient rich, high in fiber, and very low in sugar. Fruits, vegetables, and tubers are paleo friendly and gluten free, and they include foods like yams, sweet potatoes, white potatoes, cassava, jicama, taro, and Jerusalem artichokes (buy organically grown produce in this category; nonorganic potatoes and yams are genetically modified). Neocarbs are the love child of agricultural "progress": processed grains, flour products, and sugar. Twinkies didn't grow on trees, you know! It can easily be argued that neocarbs are the cause of heart disease, diabetes, autoimmune conditions, crooked teeth, shortened stature, osteoporosis, depression, and anxiety, to name a few. So when you want your carb fix, start dragging your knuckles on the ground, grunting, sniffing, and foraging around for the natural kind; sweet potatoes, winter squash, vegetables, and fresh fruit are your best options. Brown rice, beans and legumes, millet, amaranth, quinoa, steel-cut oats, buckwheat (kasha), and farro are next in line; white rice, bread, and pasta are most definitely at the bottom of the list.

Gorgeous Superfoods

Sometimes a food is more than a food. Sometimes food rises above and beyond the call of duty, armed with superpowers that quench free radicals in the body and fight aging, helping us look and feel gorgeous! I'm going to list my top five favorite superfoods to incorporate into your diet as much as possible:

- **Blueberries:** Loaded to the gills with antioxidants, these berries are the only food proven to prevent age-related memory decline. Eat at least 1 cup/150 g blueberries daily when in season; you can also buy fresh-frozen ones and add them to oats or smoothies during the winter months.
- **Cruciferous vegetables:** Brussels sprouts, cauliflower, and broccoli reign as the queens of greens because they contain indoles that prevent cancer and glutathione compounds that carry out detoxification reactions. This enables your liver to remove toxic by-products (alcohol, heavy

metals, pesticides, and so on) efficiently and effectively. Kale and Brussels sprouts help the liver perform the job of detoxification, rendering harmful substances into waste products that the body can eliminate. Don't forget fresh green juices like wheatgrass, barley grass, buckwheat, and alfalfa, which contain chlorophyll to help bind toxins and decrease cellular damage. Shred 'em and steam 'em, roast 'em, or boil and mash 'em with some olive oil and sea salt—but eat 1 to 2 cups/90 to 180 g at least three times per week for the most protective benefits.

- **Ground flaxseeds:** I'm a huge fan of ground flaxseeds because they detoxify estrogen in the liver and help prevent breast, colon, and prostate cancer. They are fiber rich, too; 2 tbsp have 6 g fiber. You can also enjoy high-lignan flaxseed oil, which has some of the same benefits. Men can also enjoy ground flaxseeds but should avoid flax oil due to its ability to raise PSA.

- **Pomegranates:** Packed with fiber (0.4 oz/11 g per serving), these sensual, tangy red bombs are rich in punicalagins, a potent antioxidant that is two to three times higher in antioxidants than red wine and green tea. The high polyphenol content in pomegranates is greater than in blueberries and cranberries, which makes them one helluva disease fighter. Drinking 4 oz/120 ml of pomegranate juice daily fights atherosclerosis and prostate cancer, helps treat active diarrhea, boosts immune function (especially when taken at the onset of a cold), and is a good tool to keep in your cancer-fighting arsenal. To enjoy fresh, whole pomegranates, score the top both lengthwise and crosswise. Over a bowl of water, hold the sides and gently use your thumb to push out the arils to the bottom of the bowl. Drain the water and serve. Arils keep up to 1 week in the fridge.

- **Sweet potatoes:** Does nature make a candy in spud form? You betcha! Rich in beta-carotene and vitamin A, potassium, and fiber (especially if you eat the skin), sweet potatoes fight inflammation, promote healing, boost lung health, reduce bodily harm from exposure to heavy metals, and are low on the glycemic index. Slice in half, place facedown in a glass pan, and bake at 375°F/190°C for 1 hour. Swipe them with some olive, flax, or coconut oil or butter to boost your absorption of beta-carotene.

Got Cravings?

What's the best way to deal with sugar cravings? For some people, it's easiest to give in to them and get them over with. But if you're trying to reach a fitness goal, this can sabotage your efforts. So here are some quick, strategic tricks that can nip those pesky cravings in the bud:

1. Make sure you are eating enough protein at each meal. Protein stabilizes blood sugar and controls the release of insulin, a potentially fat-storing hormone. If you're still hungry after meals, add in a little more protein and see if that helps.

2. Eat adequate fiber at meals by filling at least 50 percent of your plate with vegetables (raw or cooked). Have a piece of fruit for dessert.

3. Eat five or six small meals per day, and do not let more than 3 or 4 hours pass between meals. If your cravings occur in the mid-afternoon, it usually means that you ate too many carbs for breakfast and not enough protein. Protein is the only nutrient that turns off hunger signals in the brain, so eat it first at meals.

4. If you're really jonesing for a treat and the craving won't quit, stir 1 tbsp/5 g cocoa powder into warm almond milk and sweeten with stevia, or eat 1 tsp peanut butter. That should do the trick.

Crave Busters

Try incorporating these foods into your diet regularly to blast your cravings into oblivion. They will also help destroy cravings when you feel them coming on.

- Protein bars. I love Power Crunch bars, which are low-carb and soy- and gluten-free. Standard Process and Biogenesis also make great bars.
- Protein shake. You can toss a banana or a handful of frozen berries in a blender with 1 cup/240 ml almond milk, 1 scoop whey protein, 1 tsp peanut butter, 1 tsp cinnamon, 1 tbsp cocoa powder, and lots of ice.
- 2 oz/55 g fresh turkey or turkey jerky
- 1 tbsp peanut butter on a banana
- 1 cup/225 g Greek yogurt with ½ scoop whey protein, and stevia or honey to sweeten

- A handful of nuts and an apple
- Frozen cherries blended with 1 scoop chocolate whey protein and enough water and ice to make a cool, slushy treat!
- Two dried figs and 1 oz/28.5 g cheese

Done the Deed?

What if you want to indulge and have that creamy piece of chocolate cake? You can offset some of the potential damage by eating your sweet treat at the end of a meal rather than on an empty stomach; this will blunt the spikes in blood sugar. I do recommend that you schedule your favorite treats once per week (give me a martini with olives and I'm good to go), in order to keep yourself on track the rest of the week. Pleasure is a nutrient, and it's hard to maintain a clean diet when there's no fun in sight at the end of the road!

On the Road

Speaking of being on the road, let's talk about some preemptive moves you can make to set yourself up for success when you travel. First and foremost, setting your intent is crucial to being successful. Stock up on protein bars, measure out mini self-sealing bags full of protein powder and nuts and seeds, turkey or beef jerky, cocoa powder, and tea bags, and fill up your vitamin case with your supplements (I have two—one for morning and one for nighttime supplements). If you're going to rent a car at your final destination, research online what grocery or health food stores are closest to your location so you can pick up bottled water and fresh snacks. I know some fitness professionals who travel with a portable mixer like the Magic Bullet for protein shakes on the road; if you feel so inclined, go for it! Skip the airplane food if possible; it can leave you bloated and constipated. Rather than throw in the towel and leave your eating choices up to chance, treat your meals like a big adventure and forage for lean-body foods instead! When it comes to eating out in restaurants, order protein- and veggie-centric meals and treat carbs as a condiment.

At Home

Did you know that eating at home instead of restaurants and preparing your own meals can literally save your life? When you cook at home, using pure, simple ingredients free of hydrogenated oils, high-fructose corn syrup, preservatives, dyes, chemicals, salt, and poor-quality fats will give your body the nutrition it needs to keep your metabolism running smoothly and your energy up. Plus, you'll have much greater control over your portion size, so you can control the calories coming in. With one in five Americans eating breakfast at McDonald's every day, I think we can all do better for ourselves! I always hear my clients tell me that they "don't have time to cook," yet they seem to know the storyline of every prime-time TV show out there. The fact is that we do have the time; the issue is whether we use our time on things that matter. Dedicate 2 hours per week to grocery shopping, either in person or online, and at least 3 hours per week to meal preparation. When you cook, do so in bulk so you can enjoy leftovers for lunch the next day or freeze them for later use. There's nothing like having a sick day and pulling out homemade chicken soup you've been storing in the freezer for that very reason!

Need a Quickie?

For a quick meal fix, try these simple low- or no-cook solutions. Bonus: All are gluten free, too!

- A can of wild Alaskan salmon in olive oil, ¼ avocado, and a dollop of hummus, served over a bed of prewashed spinach in a bag
- Protein smoothie: 1 cup/240 ml water, 1 scoop whey protein, 1 tsp cinnamon, 1 banana, 1 tsp peanut butter. Blend with ice and serve immediately.
- A can of low-sodium vegetable soup with frozen broccoli dumped in, canned chicken in olive oil
- Turkey burgers: Mix 1 lb/455 g ground turkey with 1 tbsp dried parsley and 1 tsp onion powder; shape into flat patties and bake in Pyrex dish at 375°F/190°C for 12 minutes or until the patties reach desired doneness. Serve with salsa, avocado slices, cherry tomatoes, and steamed green beans or a green salad. Turkey burger patties can be made ahead of time and stored in the freezer.

- Egg salad: Boil 3 eggs for 11 minutes. Immediately place in an ice-water bath until completely cool. Remove eggs from shells and mash with 2 tsp olive oil or mayonnaise and 1 tsp mustard; eggs should have a finely chopped consistency when finished. Serve inside a fresh bell pepper, cut in half crosswise, with carrot and celery sticks.
- In a small saucepan, heat ¼ cup/20 g dry oat bran or buckwheat with ½ cup/120 ml water. Boil over medium-high heat until it thickens; remove from heat and stir in 1 tsp cinnamon, 1 scoop vanilla whey protein powder, and a splash of almond milk.

Detox Fox

FIVE WAYS TO DETOX DAILY

1. Eat kale, broccoli, Brussels sprouts, and bitter greens. Every day.
2. Eat 4 to 6 oz/115 to 170 g protein at meals and 2 to 4 oz/55 to 115 g of protein at snacks.
3. Eat freshly ground flaxseeds and fiber-rich fruits and vegetables every day to bind toxins and detoxify estrogen.
4. Eat natural chelators of mercury and heavy metals, such as cilantro, psyllium, garlic, and Spanish black radish.
5. Include the following supplements in your regime: 3 g glycine, 300 mg milk thistle, 300 mg lipoic acid, and 1,000 mg N.A.C. (N-acetylcysteine).

Adding It All Up

Not seeing results even while keeping a food log? You have options. First of all, make sure you are eating three meals and two or three snacks per day. If you are eating healthfully (in other words, no processed foods) and are still not losing weight, try this weight-loss trick: For 4 weeks eat fruits and vegetables in place of your starch, along with 4 to 6 oz/115 to 170 g protein and 1 to 2 tbsp fat at each meal. This helps your body shed water, fat, and excess weight—especially around the midsection. Most people feel better when they reduce grains in their diet, and everyone feels better when they avoid wheat and gluten. You should notice improvement in your digestion, skin complexion, energy level, and leanness. After 4 weeks, begin eating $^1/_3$ cup/25 g dry oat bran at breakfast and see how you do. You can gradually add back two servings of a complex starch per day for weight maintenance.

Is Your Food Having an Identity Crisis?

If a food has more than five ingredients, it's probably processed. The average "healthy" protein bar has twenty-three ingredients, and the first four include fructose and glucose syrup, with sugar following closely. Remember, if you can't ID it, don't eat it! You are better off eating a couple of squares of dark chocolate, which has only five ingredients: milk, cocoa, liqueur, vanilla, and lecithin. Or have an apple and a schmear (roughly 1 tablespoon) of peanut butter, which will score you 1 oz/30 g of protein in the process. If you decide to eat a protein bar, scrutinize the ingredients, since they'll be going into your body!

Soy Vey!

The multibillion-dollar soy industry is one of the most controversial and inflamma-tory items in the nation's food market. Based on both scientific research and what I see in practice, I do not recommend that anyone eat soy unless it is fermented and in small amounts. I have seen more damage done to the body from eating soy than high-fructose corn syrup and hydrogenated oils, because soy is a thyroid and hormone disruptor, and the effects are not always reversible. *Every patient* I see with autoimmune and thyroid conditions has had high amounts of soy in their diets. Babies and children who ingest soy formulas and soy-based foods have issues with fertility and sexual development, as well as premature menses—which increases hormone-related cancers. I am on a mission to spread the message that soy is indeed a dangerous food and should in no way, shape, or form be a regular part of anyone's diet! For the most comprehensive review on soy studies, I urge you to read *The Whole Soy Story* by Kaayla Daniel, Ph.D. In the meantime, if you must consume soy, consume it in its fermented, organic form, like miso, *natto*, and tempeh, and use it in small amounts, like a condiment.

Non-GMO Shopping List

According to the Institute for Responsible Technology, we need to steer clear of the following genetically modified (GM) ingredients: corn, soybeans, canola, cottonseed, sugar beets, most Hawaiian papaya, and a small amount of zucchini and yellow squash.

Sugar is another ingredient to watch out for. If a nonorganic product made in North America lists "sugar" as an ingredient (and does not indicate that it's pure cane sugar), then it is almost certainly made from a combination of sugar cane and GM sugar beets.

Examine your dairy products carefully as well. Products may be from cows that have been injected with GM bovine growth hormone. If it's not labeled organic or "Non-GMO Project Verified," look for labels such as "No rBGH, rBST, or artificial hormones." The American Academy of Environmental Medicine reported that "Several animal studies indicate serious health risks associated with GM food," including infertility, immune problems, accelerated aging, faulty insulin regulation, and changes in major organs and the gastrointestinal system. Please refer to the articles in the "Resources" section for more information on GMOs.

GM-Uh-Oh

There are some simple steps you can take to help yourself navigate the increasingly complex maze of choices with regard to GM foods. Buying organically grown food is a good start, as is buying products with a "Non-GMO Project Verified" seal. The same goes for baby foods and baby formulas; they must be organic in order to avoid exposure to GM foods. Buy organic juices; if you indulge in a soda, look for one made with cane sugar, because the corn syrup is inevitably a GM food. When it comes to candy, chocolate, and sweeteners, organic products with 100 percent cane sugar are the way to go. Snack foods are contraband unless organic; they use the most GM corn, soy, and oils. For condiments, oils, dressings, and spreads, choose pure olive, coconut, sesame, and grapeseed oils. Also choose jams and ice creams that are made with organic ingredients and cane sugar. The list goes on and on—you can even find non-GMO pet foods and supplements; visit www.nongmoshoppingguide.com for the whole can o' beans.

Market Value

When you're buying produce at the market, less is more. Buying less and shopping twice instead of once per week saves waste and, more important, encourages us to use fruits and vegetables while they're fresh and retain as much nutrient content as possible. Plus, fresh foods taste fabulous and look gorgeous, too! If you don't have time to get to a market that often, order groceries online and stock your freezer with frozen organic veggies, soups, stews, meats, poultry, seafood, and, yes, even guacamole. If you live along the northeast corridor in the United States you can also use www.urbanorganics.com or www.suburbanorganics.com to have fresh, organic produce delivered right to your door! Most cities around the country have organic produce delivery services; check online for options in your city.

Best Bets

If you're trying for a lean body, then you should be eating at least 75 percent of your vegetables and fruits from the lower-sugar category. The best time to enjoy higher-sugar options is within the hour after you work out, when your body can easily burn them off. Bear in mind that any one of these, regardless of when you eat it, is better than a candy bar or potato chips, so don't stress out if you don't follow this list to a tee!

LOW-SUGAR VEGETABLES
Alfalfa sprouts

Asparagus

Avocado

Bamboo sprouts

Bean sprouts

Beet greens

Bell pepper (sweet green)

Broccoli

Brussels sprouts

Cabbage

Cauliflower

Celeriac (celery root, knob celery)

Celery

Collard greens

Cucumber

Dandelion greens

Eggplant

Endive

Escarole

Garlic (1 clove)

Kale

Leek

Lettuce

Mung bean sprouts

Mushroom

Mustard greens

Okra

Onion

Radish

Red-leaf chicory (arugula)

Romaine

Shallot

Spaghetti squash

Spinach

Summer squash

String beans

Swiss chard

Tomato

Turnip greens

Watercress

Zucchini

HIGH-SUGAR VEGETABLES

Why are carrots listed in both categories? Carrot juice is high in sugars (about 5 g), while cooked carrots are low (about 3 g). Raw carrots are the lowest in sugar. Even if you were to live dangerously and eat corn and peas on the same day, it wouldn't spell disaster. French fries are another story, though!

Beets

Carrots

Corn

Parsnips

Peas

Plantains

Potatoes in all forms

Winter squash (particularly acorn and butternut)

LOW-SUGAR FRUITS

Apples

Apricot

Berries

Cherries

Fresh figs

Grapefruit

Peaches

Pears

HIGH-SUGAR FRUITS

Dried fruits

Grapes

Guava

Mango

Melon

Papaya

Pineapple

She says: I'm so addicted to coffee. It makes me happy and helps me power through my mornings—especially when I haven't slept well the night before. Must I give it up to get in shape?

E says: This question has more swing votes among health-care experts than the state of Ohio! Why the coffee controversy? Because although coffee does contain antioxidants and often facilitates digestion, it also elevates the stress hormone cortisol and hardens your arteries. Since I'm all about balance, I'll offer some pointers to you junkies out there who can't live without your fix. First, drink only 8 oz/240 ml per day. Second, drink it black or with So Delicious Unsweetened Coconut Milk Beverage to minimize the insulin spike from added dairy products. Third, drink organic coffee. Fourth, drink it unsweetened or with stevia powder. Last, to boost the nutrient content of your coffee, feel free to add 1 tbsp unsweetened organic cocoa powder and a dash of cinnamon, which helps drive insulin into cells and is loaded with phytonutrients that do a body good. My personal favorite morning bevvie is a heaping 1 tbsp cocoa powder in 12 oz/360 ml hot water with a dash of cinnamon.

She says: I'm a sugarholic and crave it every day—especially in the late afternoon and evenings. What can I do to offset these cravings?

E says: It's all about planning ahead. Sugar cravings are often the rebound effect of not eating enough early on in the day and not eating regularly enough throughout the day. Make sure you're eating five or six times per day and that you're getting protein at each meal. Eggs and oats at breakfast, a smoothie with whey protein and almond milk for a morning snack, salad with chicken for lunch, turkey slices for an afternoon snack, and a bison burger with sautéed spinach for dinner will level out your blood sugar and help offset those cravings. Also, make sure you're drinking cocoa once or twice a day by mixing 1 tbsp in 8 to 12 oz/240 to 360 ml hot water (add stevia to sweeten if necessary). Cocoa raises dopamine and serotonin levels in the brain, blasting sugar cravings into oblivion; 1 tsp cinnamon mixed in will only enhance this effect.

She says: I have been doing some research and I am confused about how alcohol can increase your belly fat. As far as I can tell from research, no scientists have been able to make a clear link between alcohol and belly fat. I understand that when the body is metabolizing alcohol, it cannot metabolize fat, so that could be a cause of weight gain—or people make worse choices when drinking alcohol, which could also lead to weight gain—but I haven't found any studies that prove that drinking alcohol will result in belly fat. Could you please lead me to your source as I try to get to the bottom of this?

E says: Alcohol has 7 calories per gram, and, although it doesn't contain any fat, it's metabolized as fat in the liver. Wear and tear on the liver can slow down your body's ability to burn fat and eliminate toxins, and ultimately to lose weight. For many folks, there's a genetic component; though some people can drink and still lose weight, most are not so lucky. So, in a nutshell, you cannot get lean by drinking alcohol. Does that mean that you'll automatically gain weight while drinking alcohol? Not necessarily—but it won't help, either. In my practice, I have found this to be true, and I've found it to be true among professional athletes as well.

She says: I am a vegetarian, and I have read in your books that, for various reasons, you believe humans must consume animal protein. Of course, non-meat eaters must supplement their diet with B_{12}, but that alone does not negate it as a potential vehicle to superior health. Frankly, the meat most people consume is packed with antibiotics and steroids and comes from animals who have suffered horrific lives in torturous conditions. It seems to me that eating an organic, high-green, full-o'-beans vegan diet and popping a small B_{12} tab is preferable to consuming the flesh or excretions of fellow beings. I myself have consumed no meat for thirty-three years, and no animal products for twenty-one years, and my doctor tells me from my blood work that I have a low to zero risk of heart disease.

E says: I appreciate your discussion about vegetarians; I myself used to be a vegetarian as well. But here's the thing: As a practitioner, I have yet to see a healthy vegetarian come into my practice. After eighteen years of experience, I can tell you that *every single one* of the female vegetarians I see are deficient in vitamin D, have poor thyroid function and/or autoimmune conditions, are frequently constipated, have dry skin, often suffer from depression, and often have irregular or no periods. My male vegetarian clients tend to fare better, but it seems clear that women often require some animal protein to support liver function and hormonal balance. I do a tremendous amount of research on a daily basis, but I must also go by what I see in practice.

I agree that animals can be inhumanely raised, but they can also be raised under humane, sustainable circumstances. For example, one of my favorite seafood sources is www.vitalchoice.com, and a favorite source of beef is www.vermontgrass fedbeef.com for grass-fed beef, which has more omega-3s than fish. Don't forget to give buffalo a whirl, since it's free of hormones and antibiotics. And incorporate vegetarian sources of protein in your diet as well—pea protein, rice protein, hemp protein, whey protein, raw nuts and nut butters, and beans and rice are all good animal-free protein sources. You may also want to read *The Whole Soy Story* by Kaayla Daniel, PhD. (www.wholesoystory.com), which mentions every single study ever published on soy. I respect your beliefs and your personal choices. The bottom line is that no one diet is right for everyone, and each person has to do what's right for him or her.

She says: Every once in a while I hear people say that fruits contain too many carbs. And carrots turning into sugar—WTF? I always thought it was good to eat more fruits and veggies!

E says: I know it sounds crazy, but yes, fruits do contain natural sugars that can impede your ability to reach your fat-loss goals if you eat too many of them. The same goes for carrots and other starchy vegetables like corn, lima beans, parsnips, and potatoes. I'm all about the spectrum of things: The fruits lowest in sugar include grapefruit, berries, apples, and pears, and the higher-sugar fruits include bananas, mangoes, pineapple, and watermelon. The vegetables lowest in sugar include kale, Brussels sprouts, broccoli, zucchini, and eggplant, and the higher-sugar vegetables include beets, carrots, parsnips, peas, and plantains. All of these fruits and vegetables have cancer- and heart disease–fighting compounds, so enjoy especially the higher-sugar fruits and vegetables earlier in the day or within the hour after finishing your workout, when your body can easily burn them off and build muscle during the temporary spike in insulin. See pages 29–31 for a comprehensive guide of low- and high-sugar fruits and vegetables.

She says: I have a desk job that is boring. How do I fight the boredom of sitting for those long, dull hours without eating M&M's or other junk food?

E says: It's all about setting your intent. The bottom line is that temptation is around us at all times; our daily challenge lies in reminding ourselves of our goals and how bad we feel when we give in to sin. Like many things in life, the fantasy of short-term pleasure is often better than the reality of the aftermath. Start creating accountability by keeping a food log—especially when you are at work. The power of the pen works wonders at turning "won't power" into willpower! Put cues in place that signal when a meal is over, like brushing your teeth or popping a breath mint, or brewing yourself a cup of peppermint tea. Think of ways to combat your at-work boredom, like going for a quick stroll, rewriting your résumé for your dream job, doing some deep-breathing exercises, or reading some interesting articles. Even taking a quick run up and down the stairwell in your office will help offset your boredom-related cravings—and it will give your energy a boost, too! Don't forget to give yourself a reward for every week you fight the candy temptation, like a manicure, a magazine, an extra-long workout, or anything else that pleases her royal thighness.

Chapter Two

GORGEOUSLY FIT

Eating and exercising for fat loss encompasses activities and diet that controls carbohydrate intake, blood sugar response, and cortisol levels—which all impact and control the hormonal effects of food. In other words, eating right to lean out is all about timing; you've got to light the metabolic fire at the right times. So if you're trying to burn fat, then you should consume high-glycemic carbs within 10 to 30 minutes of finishing your workout. Doing so is actually anabolic because insulin sensitivity is highest after a workout. And, you should pair your exercise with protein to repair muscles and support growth. Diet will control 80 percent of your body composition; exercise is the remaining 20 percent. To keep you on track and reach your fitness goals, get your body fat tested weekly. It is a far more accurate reading of your wellness than a scale. And keep reading through the entries in this chapter for more tips on melting body fat. Have fun!

Questionable Cardio

When clients come to me for weight loss, their story is often the same: "I eat healthfully and exercise but I still can't lose weight!" Change is hard, but it's also a good thing to keep things fresh by breathing new life into old, stale routines. The women I see in my practice tend to rely heavily on cardio to keep themselves in shape, yet they are frustrated at seeing little to no change in their body shape. Ladies, we *all* need to lift heavy weights to create hormonal changes within our bodies. Lifting heavy weights raises the body's levels of testosterone, human growth hormone (HGH), and dihydroxyandrosterone (DHEA). This in turn boosts the body's natural ability to burn fat for a full 24 hours after your workout! Bear in mind that eating healthy, whole foods must accompany your workouts, lest you sabotage all of your gorgeous efforts at the gym.

Lift Heavy to Get Lean

Think that it's different for girls when it comes to weight-lifting? Think that women should "tone up" by doing many reps with light weights? Think again! Considering the fact that women have lower testosterone levels than men and ultimately more challenges building muscle than men, we must replace these misconceptions about exercise and the female body with the hard truths (pun intended) about muscle. Testosterone is the anabolic hormone that contributes to increased muscle mass. Building muscle increases the amount of receptor sites for insulin, which controls your blood sugar and belly fat and ultimately facilitates fat loss in the body. And, for every 1 lb/0.5 kg of muscle you gain, you burn an extra 50 calories per day. According to my favorite strength coach, Charles Poliquin, for every 1 kilogram of lean tissue gained, there is an equal loss of weight in body fat, which can dramatically change your entire body composition. Women who lift heavy weights and really get their heart rate up during those exercises will burn up to nine times more calories during the course of the day than they would doing a cardio workout alone! Next time you're lifting weights, try adding 5 lb/2.2 kg to your load. I think you'll like what you see in the mirror.

How Much Time to Do the Crime?

I go to the gym and see the same people there day in and day out, doing the exact same routines for years and not changing their bodies one bit. What a waste of valuable time! An effective gym workout is done for 1 hour at most, three or four times per week. In addition, avoid prolonged cardio that keeps your heart rate continuously elevated at 60 to 85 percent of your maximum heart rate; this type of cardio is extremely detrimental to fat loss, because it raises cortisol levels in the body. Cortisol is a stress hormone that helps the body store fat while simultaneously burning muscle—especially around your midsection. To help build endurance and keep your heart fit, try high-intensity interval training (HIIT) for 20 to 30 minutes at a stretch, and no more than that. You will burn twice the body fat during your workouts, and the effect will last throughout the entire day. A 5-minute warm-up can be followed by five rounds of 1-minute sprints, with 30 to 60 seconds of rest in between. Then cool down for 5 minutes. Sprints can be done on a treadmill, bike, or elliptical trainer; with a jump rope; or even as fast laps in a pool. Still not convinced that HIIT will be effective? Look at the physique of a marathoner versus that of a sprinter and tell me who has more muscle!

Mix and Match

If you're starting to feel like a hamster on a wheel, doing the same weight and cardio routines for months (or even years) at a time, it's time to snap out of it! First of all, doing the same exercises repeatedly will not change your body. Your body will wise up to your antics very quickly by maintaining your fitness levels and making no strength or muscle gains whatsoever. Second, in order to build muscle, you have to break it down first by creating micro tears within the muscle tissue. This is what happens when you challenge your body by lifting heavy weights; your muscles will tear and repair themselves, a process that ultimately builds new muscle fibers. And you'd better get used to it, because once your body learns the pleasure and potency of strength gains, you'll never go back to the same useless exercises again. The other real benefit to all this, of course, is that switching out old, tired workouts for new and interesting moves lets you become the ultimate hamster on the wheel (or at least the one I'd like to be)—the one doing cartwheels!

Plyometrics

What in the world are plyometrics, you ask? They are yet another tool you can pull from your glitter-encrusted tool belt when fighting the good fight against fat. Plyometrics are explosive, fast movements that build maximum power in functional movements (sounds like sex, right?). Interspersing plyos with short recovery breaks enables the muscle to reach maximal force in the shortest possible amount of time. A typical routine might include three or four sets of fifteen squat jumps, fifteen split squats, ten bench jumps, and ten squat thrusts. Do these exercises consecutively, rest for 30 to 60 seconds, and then repeat three or four times. (Check out videos online to make sure your form is spot-on.) Incorporating these exercises into your routine will ignite your metabolic spark, making you stronger and more toned while frying calories even when you're not active. This will keep your metabolism cooking on high speed so you can burn off the occasional cookie or beer. Sign me up!

Post-Workout Muscle Mocktail

Immediately after your workout, drink 20 g BCAA in a glass of water to relieve sore muscles. Then add:

Magnesium glycinate (400 mg) with food

CoQ10 (200 mg) with food

$\frac{1}{2}$ tsp topical magnesium applied behind the knees

Repletion protein shake: 1 tbsp L-glutamine powder, 1 to 2 scoops whey protein, 1 cup/150 g berries, 1 scoop greens powder, 1 cup/240 ml water, 1 tsp cinnamon, stevia to sweeten. Blend with ice.

Fitting It All In

One of the greatest challenges of working out is actually getting to the gym. So what happens when you feel you can't get there due to work or travel commitments? Don't go! Create your own 10-minute home workout instead, which will still have your buns burning and your lungs working. Better yet, you don't need any equipment whatsoever. For 10 minutes, complete five sets of the following:

> 30 seconds squat jumps
>
> 30 seconds switch jumps
>
> 30 seconds squat thrusts
>
> 30 seconds REST

Repeat five times total to complete a 10-minute circuit. You will be dying by the end, I promise—and mighty sore afterward, too! If you have another 10 minutes, alternate 1 minute of jumping rope with 1 minute of rest until time is up. And then, if you have another 10 minutes, repeat the first exercise circuit. For online visuals of the exercises above and more workout ideas, pick up *My Gym Trainer* by Jill Coleman at www.mytrainerfitness.com or go to www.metaboliceffect.com for personally tailored online workouts.

Exercise: Your Metabolic Modulator

Think that 30 minutes of intense exercise isn't as effective as an hour on the treadmill? Think again! If you're starved for time in your day, you may not have the time for an hour workout, anyway (I know I don't!). Think of exercise like sex: how hard you do it may be even more important than how long. Staying on the treadmill like a hamster on a wheel does burn calories but ultimately is catabolic and breaks down muscle. On the flip side, cardio-based weight training burns fat for hours and even days after you've done the deed, which means you can exercise less and burn more! And here's more good news for you: Lifting heavy weights and doing short but intense bursts of cardio naturally balances out your hormones and controls hunger and sugar cravings. It just doesn't get any better than that!

Sleep Is a Fat-Loss Nutrient

Let's face it—hormones are one helluva dominatrix when it comes to ruling our bodies. Night after night of abuse (like sleep deprivation, for example) and you'll be feeling that whip crack your booty, all right! Sleep is critical in controlling fat storage because of the role it plays in regulating our hormones. Two hormones in particular rule the roost with appetite regulation: ghrelin and leptin. Ghrelin says "I'm hungry" and leptin says "I've had enough."

Leptin decreases your appetite after you've eaten, and it promotes calorie burning. Obese people have high levels of leptin, but their bodies may be less sensitive to its effects. Ghrelin is the hunger hormone, which tells you that you need to eat. Ghrelin also contributes to stress eating, and you can blame it for your high-calorie food cravings and the abdominal fat you're storing. It's no surprise that eating meats and nuts in your meals controls ghrelin, while eating sugary snacks will spike it. And, research from the University of Chicago says that sleep deprivation increases ghrelin, decreases leptin, and increases the incidence of obesity. In other words, a few extra hours of shut-eye are imperative in fighting the battle of the bulge. Read on to learn how you can improve the quality and duration of your sleep through gorgeous lifestyle choices.

Cortisol Cowgirl

No discussion of workouts and getting lean would be complete without a chat about cortisol. I keep mentioning it, but what is it, how does it work in the body, and how can you manage it? If you play your cards right, cortisol can work for you and help you build lean muscle. Cortisol is the primary stress hormone secreted by the adrenal glands—kind of like a low-grade adrenaline. The adrenal glands are each about the size of a walnut and enlarge during times of stress, kicking out trace minerals like magnesium and zinc, and causing you to crave stimulants like caffeine and sugar. Cortisol is secreted during the stress response, but it also remains elevated with lack of adequate sleep, overtraining with exercise, and skipping meals— not to mention fighting with your spouse before bed, late-night drinking and eating sweets, and realizing at eleven o'clock at night that you've forgotten to pay an overdue bill—ack! High cortisol levels cause you to store fat and burn muscle, kick your sex drive to the curb, and give you heart disease and a high gut-to-butt ratio. (When your gut sticks out farther than your butt does, you have a high gut-to-butt ratio, and you also probably have Syndrome X, which encompasses insulin resistance, high triglycerides, and high blood pressure. It's the main stop on the highway to a heart attack.) So let's discuss some strategic moves to help keep these unwanted effects in a land far, far away.

The release of cortisol is tightly regulated by the body. It peaks at about eight in the morning to help get your booty of out bed for the day. Throughout the day, cortisol levels drop off and reach their lowest levels between eight and ten o'clock at night so you can more easily travel to the land of nod. So if you are overtraining or overstressed (or even over caffeinated) and have chronically elevated cortisol levels, your chances of tossing and turning all night like a rotisserie chicken are pretty high. The good news is that a few strategic moves can get you sleeping like you just had a whopper orgasm and then conked out after. (Did I mention that sex ain't a bad way to combat insomnia, either?)

To be the mistress of your own domain when it comes to cortisol, try these helpful tips:

- Eat within an hour of waking up, and eat at regular intervals throughout the day, since skipping meals elevates cortisol.
- Keep your carb intake in check; eating too many carbs and elevating your insulin levels will signal your body to release cortisol into your bloodstream.
- Start shutting down for the night by 9:30 P.M. to facilitate the release of restorative hormones and ensure a good night's sleep.
- Breathe to lower your cortisol. Any time of day is effective, but doing deep-breathing exercises before bed can break the vicious cycle of anxiety and insomnia. All you need is 10 minutes.
- Steer clear of stimulants like ephedra and caffeine, because they will turn on your "fight or flight" response and send you into overdrive. Some people take 24 hours to clear one cup of morning caffeine from their systems. No caffeine should pass your lips after 2:00 P.M. if you're having trouble sleeping!
- Limit workouts to 60 minutes (unless you are walking, which will lower your cortisol). With nonwalking workouts, at the 60-minute mark, your testosterone levels start to decline and cortisol levels rise—not a good combo.

She says: How can I get motivated to get to the gym? I put the gym at the bottom of my list, when it really should be first! It's so hard to get to the gym when I don't get home until after seven at night, and by then I'm starving and just want to chill! How can I get a workout in, or keep up my energy levels so I'm not fading at the end of the day?

E says: Not to worry, my worker bee—you *can* have it all! Thank heavens for the paradigm shift in exercise physiology, because less is truly more when it comes to working out. Even professional bodybuilders do not spend more than an hour working out at a time, so I'm confident you can get your fix in 20 to 30 minutes. I suggest that you get up 45 minutes earlier to squeeze in a workout first thing in the morning, on an empty stomach—you'll burn 30 percent more fat in doing so. (If you feel better with some food in your stomach before a workout, then add $^1\!/_2$ to 1 scoop of whey protein or 5 g BCAAs in 8 oz/240 ml water and drink it down— ideally 30 minutes before a workout.) And you'll check it off your to-do list nice and early, before the day gets away from you. Warm up by jumping rope for 5 minutes; then grab a dumbbell and incorporate some plyometrics into your regime. Do three or four sets of the following while holding a medium-weight dumbbell, twelve reps each set: walking lunges, squat thrusts, dead lifts, and dumbbell squat jumps. Wear a heart-rate monitor to make sure you see a rise in your heart rate during sets; you should be breathless and sweaty by the end of the first set. Rest in between as needed, but only rest until you recover—ideally no more than 30 seconds—then get right back to it. Do this three times per week, and walk on the weekends for at least an hour. If you have time, take walks during the week, too; walking helps lower stress hormones and will balance out the high intensity of your plyometrics. Be sure to check out the "Lean-Body Diet" (see pages 120–125) for ideas on how to struc-ture your eating to help optimize your energy before and after workouts, and see page 70 for supplements that alleviate post-workout soreness. And don't forget to get in bed by 9:30 P.M. so you can rise and shine the next morning!

She says: I've heard that the best advantage you can give yourself in your workouts is a great night's sleep, and that lights should be out by ten o'clock for optimal adrenal function and endurance—especially if you're doing sprints or lifting heavy weights. Can you give me some tips to help myself fall asleep?

E says: Meditation and deep breathing, topical and oral magnesium to relax and repair muscles, and some Yogi Bedtime Tea are also great for an overactive mind. I keep the lights low, drop the temperature, get away from the computer and TV, and think about the healthy aspects of adequate sleep. You can also try the Lumie light, which slowly turns off at night and slowly lights up in the morning before the alarm goes off. Lovely! It helps combat seasonal affective disorder, too. Don't forget to count your blessings by thinking of at least three positive things you have seen, done, or felt during the day.

She says: I always seem to struggle with working out consistently. Interrupted sleep, travel, and stress leave me fatigued the next day and make exercise such a challenge! What are some strategies you can recommend to help me stay on track, with or without a workout?

E says: I used to adhere to the all-or-nothing attitude in my workouts until I changed the way I work out. The truth is that you can have just as effective a workout in 20 minutes as you can with a 60-minute stint on the treadmill. First and foremost, numerous studies have shown that sprinting, alternating with 1-minute rest periods, burns 30 percent more fat than doing an hour of cardio. Plus, it takes half the time to do your workouts and you burn fat for twice as long afterward! You can also do 20 to 30 minutes of weight circuits by alternating lifting heavy weights with squat jumps, walking lunges, 1-minute sprints on the treadmill, or jumping rope. The goal is to have your heart rate spike at intervals throughout your workouts. The foundation beneath all of this is, of course, a healthy diet, because you may not see any change in your body at all if you do not change what you put in it. Ask not what you can do to your food, but what your food can do to you!

Chapter Three

FEELING GORGEOUS

We must remember that *pleasure* is a nutrient. It's important to balance out our clean eating with indulgences. A diet of whole foods will keep your immune system, bones, muscles, and skin happy and healthy! So much of our time is dedicated to counting calories without ever considering what foods we actually want to eat and what our bodies enjoy eating. Consequently, eating can become an uninspired chore. Before you pop a mindless bite into your mouth, ask yourself what you *truly* want to eat. Something hot or cold? Liquid or solid? Crunchy or chewy? Sweet, sour, or salty? Turning mindless eating into mindful eating will give you a level of satisfaction that will ultimately allow you to transcend cravings, junk food, and overeating, and help you recover the joy of one of the greatest sensory pleasures on this heavenly Earth!

Pearls of Wisdom

My late mentor Robert Crayhon gave me so many clinical pearls of wisdom that I still cherish today. One of them is this: You should eat foods for what they do have, rather than for what they don't have. You want to eat a food that has the right essential fatty acids, not because it's fat free. The same goes for "natural" foods, a moniker that is often abused on product labels. Robert used to say, "Gasoline is natural, but I wouldn't tell you to drink it!" In an age when so much is available to us at the click of a keypad, we owe it to ourselves to think critically so that we may eat gorgeously. Rather than taking claims at face value, let's bring out the conspiracy theorist within all of us and question our food and the motives behind the choices we make.

Black or White?

Is eating a black-and-white choice for you? Do you feel that if you indulge at one meal it's all downhill for the rest of the day, or do you just put yourself back on track at the next meal? So much of how we act and interact with food is based on our perception of ourselves. If we feel good about ourselves, we eat gorgeously. So toss out your scale and your inner critic and focus on the progress you make each day through eating well and exercising. Buy clothes that highlight your assets, even if it means going up one or two sizes for the time being. No matter what size you are, you deserve to look and feel fabulous. And, ultimately, your clothes will be a better (and more fun) way to measure how your body is changing.

Lone Star

Never let weakness convince you that you lack strength. Eating clean goes against mainstream Western culture and therefore it takes courage to do so. When it comes to setting goals, focus on doing things that make you feel good about yourself and that give you a sense of accomplishment each day: Buying nutritious foods and working out are my personal faves. Often, we wait to be inspired when it's really our responsibility to inspire others—so become the inspiration you've always sought. Living gorgeously is really about progress, not perfection.

Skin-tastic

I often train professionals in the beauty industry on how to provide their clients with lifestyle, diet, and supplement recommendations for skin health. So let me share the insider scoop with you. Think of your skin as your intestines turned inside out; your skin is an excellent indicator of your digestive and immune wellness. If you suffer from acne, rosacea, eczema, or inflammation, incorporate wild Alaskan salmon into your diet at least three times per week and 16 to 32 billion probiotic organisms into your daily regime. Wild Alaskan salmon is an anti-inflammatory food rich in DMAE (dimethylaminoethanol) that will quench your inner fires and help your skin glow. Probiotics will help rebalance the levels of good bacteria in your intestinal tract, reduce or eliminate food allergies, and help control acne. Don't forget to pop at least 25 mg of zinc daily to help balance your hormones and control acne outbursts.

Flu Shot? Fugeddaboudit!

In my professional opinion, the flu shot is not a necessary component of staying healthy in the winter. Beating the bugs is as simple as vitamins A, D, and C! Sweet potatoes, cantaloupe, carrots, and winter squash are in season in the winter for good reason—they contain vitamin A, which supports lung function. Generated mainly by exposure to sunlight, vitamin D is in short supply in the winter, so supplement your diet by consuming wild Alaskan salmon and cod liver oil during the dark months. Vitamin C naturally fights viruses and boosts immune function. Winter citrus fruits like oranges, grapefruits, and clementines rock the house with vitamin C, but feel free to take an additional 500 to 1,000 mg of vitamin C daily to ensure adequate levels in the body.

How to Get Your Body in Tip-Top Shape

1. Get enough sleep each night, and be consistent about it.
2. Eat organic and locally grown foods as often as possible.
3. Eat more calories during the day, when you are active, and fewer at night.
4. Lift weights three to four times per week.
5. Get your vitamin D levels checked with a 25-OH vitamin D blood test; aim for 80 to 120 ng/dL. Research currently shows that the best way to take vitamin D_3 is by administering high doses twice weekly; this could be anywhere from 10,000 to 50,000 IU at a time. If that number sounds high to you, don't worry; 10,000 IU of vitamin D is equivalent to 10 minutes in the sun without wearing sunscreen.

Climb Your Highest Mountain

Although our brains have preprogrammed, hardwired habits, they are also malleable and capable of change. That is why visualization can help us reach our goals. According to Harvard researcher Srinivasan Pillay, M.D., imagined action and actual movement activate the same parts of the brain, so by picturing your intended outcome you are giving the brain the information it needs in order to figure out your course of action. If you want to perform jumping lunges, look down and see yourself in black shorts, see the floor of the gym and your feet on it, and give yourself the feeling of performing jumping lunges. Then give those lunges a real-life try. If you're doubtful about your ability to meet your goal, tell yourself that it may be difficult but it's possible. When you think a goal is possible, that gives the brain permission to reach it!

Sparking Your Circuits

The greatest thing about having a brain is that you can retrain it and create positive changes within yourself. Meditation is one of my favorite ways to rewire oneself, because it promotes a sense of calm and relaxation all day long—even if you do it the night before. The amygdala, an almond-shaped mass of nerve cells deep in the brain that regulates our emotions, is the greatest heir of meditative benefits. Loving-kindness meditation stabilizes the amygdala, fostering compassion toward the self and others. So if you are feeling anxious, are struggling with insomnia, or just crave some deeply restorative and relaxing sleep, practice some self-love in your head, and watch the magic unfold after a few short days.

The Psychology of Change

How many psychologists does it take to change a light bulb? Only one—but it has to really want to change! Creating permanent behavior change is rarely a simple process, and requires both time and an emotional commitment. The ability to change requires a tremendous amount of support and an open path to follow. You must ask yourself if you're ready to change. Is there anything to prevent you from changing? What triggers might cause you to relapse into a former behavior? Don't be afraid to write down your goals and tell other people what you are doing— this is a powerful way to help yourself achieve success. Reward yourself for each milestone you achieve. Start small so your goals can be attainable. Develop coping strategies to deal with temptation. If you lapse, get right back on the horse! By preparing for and maintaining a new behavior, you will be more likely to succeed.

Gorgeous Revolution

When it comes to making food choices, instead of saying, "I'll be good," why not say, "I'll be good to myself"? Invest your energy in the power of positive thinking for your greatest yield on results—it works!

Five More Ways to Detox Daily

1. Drink shots of fresh wheatgrass daily, and/or drink red and green vegetable juice powder reconstituted with water.
2. Exercise and sweat out toxins.

3. Take a sauna for 10 minutes, preferably an infrared sauna, to release toxins.
4. Soak in a bath with 2 cups/500 g Epsom salts and 1 cup/220 g baking soda.
5. Breathe, meditate, let go of negative thoughts, and bring on the gratitude! Practicing yoga is extremely beneficial for this very reason.

Mind-fullness

"If you can find a path with no obstacles, it probably doesn't lead anywhere."
—Frank A. Clark

What breakthroughs have you had in your eating, exercise, or life plan that have helped you reach your personal goals? Sometimes the spark that ignites change comes when we sit down with ourselves and have some honest conversations. Paradigm shifts happen gradually, over time, but if you have good support and truly believe in and visualize your goals, you will reach them in time. You may not always see changes right away, but you must keep plugging along. One day you'll catch yourself in the mirror, and poof! A new you. Isn't life grand when your projects take shape and all your hard work becomes tangible?

The Brighter Side of Life

As I age I try to become increasingly positive and surround myself with like-minded people. So here's my gift to you: some gorgeous mantras that are calorie free yet soulfully decadent!

GORGEOUS GIRL BEFORE	GORGEOUS GIRL AFTER
I'm being "good."	I'm being good to myself.
I'm not doing enough.	I'm doing what's right for me.
I'm too tired to go to the gym.	I'm blessed to be able to work out.

Beating ourselves up for not meeting the perfect standard of thinness, muscularity, body shape, and so on is like throwing down a roadblock right in the middle of our path to success. Show those ugly voices in your head right to the door and feng shui your mind from useless clutter. Buy clothes that fit your body type, no matter what your size or age. What seems to be a flaw in your eyes may be your best attribute in someone else's. Now go and tell yourself how gorgeous and amazing you are—I dare you!

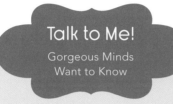

Talk to Me!
Gorgeous Minds
Want to Know

She says: What helps keep you motivated and on track when you're trying to eat well and exercise?

E says: A food log is immensely helpful because you have to be accountable and conscious of your choices. If you bite it, you write it! Having a workout partner and someone to report to also makes a difference if your motivation is down. Sometimes it's a professional like a nutritionist or personal trainer; often a friend can do the trick, too. Make sure to surround yourself with positive people who inspire you to strive to do better!

She says: How do you keep yourself motivated once the finish line (like hitting your goal weight) is near? How do you not get lazy and stop when the end is in sight?

E says: Think about why you wanted to lose the weight in the first place. Was it really just about the weight? Or has losing weight improved your life in other ways, like giving you increased energy, sex drive, and improved self-esteem? It's important to understand your motivations, because this will ensure your long-term success. To keep yourself on track is a lifelong discipline and will require some helpful tools that will hold you accountable to yourself. I really love to have clients track their weight and body fat to help them stay within their desired range. You can do this with a Tanita scale (www.tanita.com) on a weekly basis; make sure you take your measurements at the same time and day each week, and don't let yourself gain more than 5 pounds/2.25 kilograms or 2 percent body fat above your target. An unwanted change in the way your pants fit is a clear indicator that you've fallen off the wagon. Also, if you find yourself really slipping off track, like during a vacation or the holidays, start writing down what you eat. Food logs are an amazing tool for creating cognitive changes and mindfulness; for me they are a total reset button. And don't forget to put your goals on a timeline. "Lose a dress size" is a long-term goal that can easily become abstract, whereas writing down "hit the gym five times this week, lose 1 to 2% body fat, eat five times per day, and keep a food log" breaks your goal into a structured plan. Once you reach your goals and have maintained your size for a few months, have your clothes taken in or buy new ones for your smaller size. Good luck!

She says: How do I motivate to get to the gym when the weather is cold and gross and I don't want to go?!

E says: Getting to the gym is like working for the postal service; neither rain nor cold nor snow shall keep you away! Exercise requires commitment and planning—and *consistency*. Half the battle is won just by showing up! So put your blinders on and your earplugs in (weather reports will just depress you) and make going to the gym your priority, year-round, no matter what the weather. Lay out your clothes the night before, have a bottle of water and a towel ready by the front door, get in bed by 9:30 P.M., and visualize your workout the night before you do it. Print out a calendar for yourself and plan out what exercises you are going to do each day of the week—and give yourself a gold star every day you complete your goal. Once or twice a week try to meet a friend at the gym or take a group class to make it more fun and social. Nothing beats laughter and camaraderie while getting fit!

She says: I have gained weight, and now my clothes are tight, but I can't bear the thought of buying a bigger size. How can I feel prettier going out on the town with my sexy friends?

E says: To paraphrase a quote from *Sex and the City*, feeling thin is more about a state of mind than a state of behind! There are a couple of great fashion trompe l'oeil tricks you can try. First, dress monochromatically and accessorize with jewelry or scarves around your face to bring out the eyes. Do your makeup and style your hair. Dress in forgiving fabrics like jersey, and think about flattering silhouettes for your body shape. If you've got a small waist but are sporting some junk in the trunk, a wrap dress with high-heeled boots will do you justice. Or, you can cover up that muffin top with a retro flowy top and a long, streamlined cardigan. I'd encourage you to also work with a nutritionist to give you the support and guidance you need to help you shed the unwanted weight. Reading this book is a great place to start, and there are online options and phone consultations as well. But in the meantime, be good to yourself and add one or two items to your wardrobe that fit your body and help you feel beautiful.

She says: I'm turning forty-five this spring. How can that be? I see "old" in the mirror now. How do I let my inner sixteen-year-old show up on my face?

E says: Sugar, coffee, breads, pasta, and excess dairy will leave you looking saggy, haggy, dehydrated, and dull. Not such a pretty picture. But having a gorgeous face and getting your youthful groove back is much easier than you think. You need to feed your face with gorgeous, antioxidant-rich, clean foods. Think proteins like wild Alaskan salmon, chicken, egg whites, and whey protein, hypoallergenic starches like brown rice, sweet potatoes, winter squash, legumes, and mineral-rich fats like raw nuts and seeds, nut butters, coconut flakes, and avocadoes. Don't forget cantaloupe, blueberries, and pomegranates, and dark-green leafy veggies like Brussels sprouts, broccoli, spinach, and kale to plump up your skin and detoxify your liver. Glow, baby, glow! Also remember to exfoliate twice weekly with a sugar scrub: Wet your face with warm water and massage 1 tsp sugar into your skin until it dissolves into a sticky but smooth serum (1 to 2 minutes). Rinse well and pat dry; apply moisturizer. Luminous lady!

Chapter Four

GORGEOUS HEALTH AND IMMUNITY

Although sick days can be a valuable time to catch up on e-mails and watch movies, I'd rather be healthy. And while we can't kick every cold that heads our way, we now know that the right combination of supplements can shorten the duration and intensity of a cold. The trick is catching a cold right when it starts. So when you feel like you're starting to get run down, turn to this chapter for protocols and recipes that will have your white cells grooving in no time. And don't forget a girl's best friend, vitamin D_3, which is absorbed through each and every cell in our body. Tough stuff!

A Sip from the Devil's Cup?

Is too much vitamin D toxic? Absolutely. Is vitamin D toxicity rare? Abso-freakin-lutely. Your blood level of vitamin D should be 80 to 120 ng/dL. Most people need 5,000 to 10,000 IU per day (the equivalent of spending 5 to 10 minutes in the sun without sunscreen). You can also take 50,000 IU once per week if your levels are really low; high doses taken once or twice per week optimize absorption of vitamin D_3.

If you are already supplementing with vitamin D, you may need to boost your dosage; taking 5,000 IU per day will usually only raise your levels to 50 during the winter months. So if your levels are low, try taking 50,000 IU of vitamin D twice per week for 3 months and then retest your levels. In the summer months, get at least 15 to 30 minutes per day of sun exposure without sunscreen, if you can tolerate it without burning. With regular sun exposure you should not need to take as much, if any, vitamin D supplements.

Also, make sure you take 500 mcg of vitamin K_1 and 500 mcg of vitamin K_2 when you are taking your vitamin D_3; together they make a great team in keeping arteries flexible. And eat colorful vegetables and fruits to ensure you are eating enough vitamin A. Ingesting food-based vitamin A along with vitamin D promotes optimal absorption.

The Heart of the Matter

Vitamin D has a wide range of functions in the body, and ongoing research continues to shed light on its diversity and importance. For example, I find vitamin D deficiencies in many of my clients with autoimmune disease, cardiovascular disease, cancer, winter colds and flu, and seasonal affective disorder (SAD). Now here's the crazy part: A study published in August 2008 ("25-Hydroxyvitamin D Levels and the Risk of Mortality in the General Population," by Michal L. Melamed, Erin D. Michos, Wendy Post, and Brad Astor, from the *Archives of Internal Medicine*, pages 1629-1637) showed that nearly two thousand people studied for five years had a 62 percent higher incidence of cardiovascular events if they had low vitamin D status. Zoinks! So if you have any of the above symptoms, poor bone density, depression, excess body fat, and/or a family history of heart disease, get yourself on some high-dose vitamin D pronto!

D-lightful

When you're heading into the cooler winter months with reduced sun exposure, it's a great time to get your baseline vitamin D checked with a 25-OH vitamin D blood test. Optimal levels need to be 80 to 120 ng/dL. Most medical journals report that a level of 30 to 50 is "normal"—but this advice is no longer current or accurate. So critical is vitamin D to the body that the human genome contains more than twenty-seven hundred binding sites for vitamin D metabolites! Vitamin D deficiency has been implicated in at least seventeen types of cancer, as well as autoimmune diseases, heart disease and stroke, bone loss, diabetes, depression, asthma, and birth defects in newborns. Visit www.vitamindcouncil.org for the most recent information on vitamin D.

The Magnesium Trifecta

Magnesium is needed by more than three hundred enzymes in the body. Topical magnesium helps raise DHEA levels, which ultimately helps to keep you lean and your mojo going. If you're deficient in magnesium, you may be impairing your ability to synthesize DHEA in the body. Either way, both are depleted by stress, yet both help manage stress. Magnesium deficiency is common in patients with diabetes, chronic fatigue syndrome, heart arrhythmias, mitral valve prolapse, heart attacks, and asthma. To optimize your magnesium levels on a daily basis, here's what you need to do each evening:

1. Take a magnesium mixture at bedtime: combine glycinate, orotate, taurate, and fumarate for a total of 400 mg magnesium. Don't worry; this will not cause diarrhea. Instead, it will be absorbed by the muscles, gut, and brain.
2. Soak in a warm bath sprinkled with 2 to 4 cups/500 to 1,000 mg Epsom salts. Soak for at least 15 minutes to let the magnesium absorb into your skin.
3. Rub two pumps of topical magnesium cream behind each knee, where it is quickly absorbed. You can rub it into the soles of your feet, too. Topical magnesium is a great way to administer magnesium to kids, who are often deficient in magnesium due to high stress and high-sugar diets.

Magnesium should be used for people with high blood pressure, diabetes, constipation, ADD (magnesium calms the nervous system), insomnia, restless leg syndrome and leg cramps, and menstrual cramps (magnesium is a muscle relaxer). It can even be used as an occasional hangover remedy (since excess alcohol consumption leads to magnesium deficiency)! It is safe for both adults and children (start with topical use or an Epsom salts bath for children). Using it both topically and orally ensures optimal absorption without any digestive side effects. My favorite magnesium products (both topical and oral) are made by Charles Poliquin: www.charlespoliquin.com.

Itchy, Scratchy?

A sore, itchy throat and respiratory congestion are some of the more common symptoms of a cold. Simple at-home remedies for sore throats are often the best options! One such simple remedy is gargling with salt water. This seems to help for several reasons. A saline solution can draw excess fluid from inflamed tissues, reducing throat pain. Gargling also loosens thick mucus, and when mucus is removed it can take with it irritants like allergens, bacteria, and fungi from the throat. For best results, dissolve ½ tsp salt in a full glass of warm water and gargle the solution for a few seconds before spitting it out. You can also try mixing warm water with lemon and honey as a more palatable option, which you can simply enjoy as a comforting beverage; no need to spit it out.

Massive Attack

Slammed with an allergy attack? Pop 1,000 mg vitamin C, chew 1 capsule primrose oil, and chase both with 1 tsp echinacea tincture in a 1 oz/30 ml shot of pomegranate juice. Your allergies will be gone within the hour! Don't forget to stay well hydrated and chug some nettle tea to help keep allergies at bay. Contrary to popular belief, it is actually safe and effective to take echinacea for longer periods of time, especially throughout the allergy season.

Just in Case

Have you packed up your vitamins in a pill-organizing case yet? It's the most time-efficient and fail-proof way to adhere to your supplement regime. At the beginning of each week, put your daily supplements into a case with a spot for each day, labeled with product and dosages, so you can take them with you as you whiz through your day. I like to take a handful in the morning and another before bed—energizing supplements and omegas in the morning; calming, sleep-inducing, muscle-repairing nutrients at night. The thing about vitamins is this: They always work better in your body than in the bottle! Taking your vitamins has a domino-like effect; you look and feel better when you take them, have more energy, have less cravings, and are healthier from the inside out, so you're more likely to keep taking them.

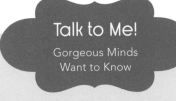

Talk to Me!
Gorgeous Minds
Want to Know

She says: Why do I have such a hard time getting rid of colds? They seem to stick around for months! And how do I avoid getting sick before going away on vacation?

E says: Being unable to kick your cold is probably a sign that you need really good sleep, a superhealthful diet, regular exercise, and some vitamins to get your body's immune system back on track. You've got a high-maintenance bod (who doesn't?), and that's not a bad thing; it just means you need to give it extra love. Clean house internally by eliminating sugar, processed and flour-based foods, and poor-quality junk foods, and replace them with whole foods rich in nutrition like fish, dark-green leafy vegetables, fresh fruits, raw nuts and seeds, and sweet potatoes. You should also consider daily juicing, either with freshly made juices or powdered green and red juices that can be reconstituted with water. Your immune system will soak up all the extra vitamins and minerals like no one's business. Exercise like walking, lifting weights, and Bikram yoga will also help elevate your white blood cell count for hours afterward, which fights infection and will ultimately resolve your cold. The following supplements can help fight the good fight against viruses and bacteria and boost your immune system overall; keep them on hand for travel as well.

Probiotics	24 billion per day
Vitamin C	1,000 mg per day
Zinc	50 mg per day for 3 months at first; 25 mg per day maintenance dose
N.A.C.	1,000 mg
Vitamin D	10,000 IU every other day for 3 months; then get your blood levels tested. Make sure your blood level is 80 to 120 ng/dL, which can be maintained by taking 10,000 IU twice per week.

She says: Is the immune system affected by probiotics?

E says: Absolutely! In fact, 60 to 70 percent of our intestinal tract is lined with lymph nodes. So if you have a healthy gut, your immune system will reap the benefits. Your intestines naturally contain 3 to 4 lb/1.35 to 1.80 kg of beneficial bacteria, helping the digestive tract and immune system stay healthy. For this reason, it's imperative that you take them during and after a course of antibiotics or antifungal medications, and while you're on oral contraceptives, so that you can replace the helpful bacteria that you lose while taking these medications. Probiotics are found in most yogurts and are available in powdered or capsule form. Probiotics are most commonly sold under the names "acidophilus," "bifidus," or "lactobacillus." Aim to take 24 billion probiotics per day, with food. And if you have food poisoning, triple that dose during the course of a day to wipe out the bad guys.

She says: Does sugar affect the immune system? I've heard it's poison—is that true?

E says: Sugar can adversely affect the immune system in so many ways. Sugar can halt white blood cell function for up to 5 hours after ingestion, putting your entire immune system on hold. Even scarier is the fact that the surface of a cancerous mass has up to ten times more insulin receptors than a regular cell in the body.

In addition, sugar raises triglyceride levels and can lead to a fatty liver. Do I think that having dessert one or two times per week is a serious problem? No. But if sugar is a part of your daily repertoire, I'd urge you to get to a nutritionist pronto to create a more balanced diet. Sugar was never a part of the hunter-gatherer diet and is now more prevalent than ever in the form of high-fructose corn syrup, super-size sodas and candy, protein bars and sports drinks, and even tomato sauces! Use it judiciously and as a special treat only.

She says: I'm just not a pill-popping gal. What are some other ways to stay healthy besides taking supplements?

E says: I love that you're thinking outside the box! There's certainly more than one way to skin a cat when you're fighting the good immune fight. Stretching is a great way to get your macrophage mojo moving. Skeletal muscle contractions help the lymphatic fluid in your body circulate more freely so you can clear waste and improve the body's ability to fight illness. Walking also stimulates lymph flow. If it's too chilly to walk outside, stretches alone will stimulate your defenses. You can also treat yourself to a massage or work with a practitioner who knows how to perform lymphatic-drainage body work. Good stuff!

Here are some lymph-loving stretches you might try:

Sore Throat Soother: Standing or sitting with chest lifted and shoulders moving down, allow your head to drop forward. Relax and hold for 30 seconds.

Cough Calmer: Place hands on the back of a chair and walk backward until your arms and spine are fully extended. Keep your legs straight and tailbone slightly lifted as you sink your spine toward the floor and allow your head to relax; hold for a minute.

Groin Girl: Lie on the floor with your sit bones against the wall and your legs pointing upward. Reach your legs up the wall and allow them to drop open as far as you can while keeping them straight and against the wall. Rest here for 1 to 2 minutes.

Chapter Five

GORGEOUS SUPPLEMENTS

Nutritional supplements can help ensure a leaner, more fabulous, healthier you! The following supplements complement the topics we've discussed in this book, and are compiled from seventeen years of practice and research. The key with supplements is the quality and the dosage; if you take poor-quality supplements and inadequate dosages, you're just wasting your time and money. Invest in yourself and your health and work with an integrative dietitian or a holistic M.D. when deciphering the best supplements for yourself. If you want even more guidance regarding what supplements to take to meet your individual goals, check out the extensive information in my first book, *Eat, Drink, and Be Gorgeous*.

Building and Repairing Muscle

An essential part of building and repairing muscles is with branched-chain amino acids (BCAAs). What are BCAAs? BCAAs are composed of the amino acids leucine, isoleucine, and valine and can be used directly by muscle tissue for energy, which is why I love to take them immediately following a workout. During intense weight training, the body's need for BCAAs is increased so it can continue to build muscle tissue. So, to increase performance, take 10 g of BCAAs before and/or after a strenuous workout; this will help replace BCAAs in the muscle, improve muscle recovery, and minimize the effects of overtraining. BCAAs not only help to make other amino acids in the body but they also improve your energy levels throughout the day. Ideally, you should take your BCAAs at a time when you are not consuming other proteins so they don't compete for absorption. Another option is to supplement with pea protein. Pea protein has an excellent array of amino acids, including high levels of BCAAs, and is extremely digestible because it is dairy- and gluten-free.

Partners in Crime

Nutrients are team-oriented workers; they always work best in conjunction with other particular nutrients, since that is how they occur in nature. To optimize the effectiveness of BCAA supplementation, you should take them with the following nutritional cofactors:

- **Chromium picolinate:** Chromium is a nutrient that increases the efficacy of insulin, a hormone composed of 91 amino acids. Insulin is the most essential link in the muscle-building chain. Chromium improves protein synthesis in the body, sweeping up free amino acids from the blood stream and helping them enter the cells. In other words, chromium helps preserve muscle. Chromium dosage: 200 to 400 mcg per day.
- **Zinc and vitamin B6:** Zinc regulates insulin and B6 is the cofactor. As athletes increase their protein intake, so should they increase vitamin B6 to help drive amino acids into the cells. Dosage: 25 mg zinc and 25 mg B6 per day.

- **Vitamin B12:** Vitamin B12 is another water-soluble nutrient that must be present in order to build muscle. B12 ensures that your brain and muscle tissue are effectively communicating, which has a direct effect on the body's ability to develop and increase muscle mass. Dosage: 1,000 mcg.
- **Biotin:** Biotin has an important role in building muscle and manufacturing glycogen. Both chromium and biotin can enhance glucose uptake in muscle and liver tissue, optimizing protein synthesis. Dosage: 2,000 mcg.

Bloat Busters

Taking B_6 and taurine together provides gentle yet effective diuretic effects so your clothes will fit you all month long!

SUPPLEMENTS

Vitamin B_6	50 mg per day
Taurine	1,000 mg per day

NUTRITIONAL APPROACHES

For diuretic benefits, drink 2 tbsp unsweetened cranberry juice diluted in 8 oz/240 ml water three times daily. Heap plenty of asparagus and sautéed dandelion greens on your plate, and enjoy a little watermelon for dessert to also help you shed extra water. Make sure you drink at least 12 glasses of water per day and eat fruits and vegetables in place of carbs for three days. Don't even think about booze—it can help you retain an extra 2 to 4 lb/0.9 to 1.8 kg of water for up to four or five days after you consume it!

Daily Detox

A healthy liver is your most important asset in cancer prevention. The protocol below will help keep your liver happy and healthy.

SUPPLEMENTS

Glycine	3,000 mg per day
Milk thistle	300 mg per day
Lipoic acid	300 mg per day
N.A.C.	1,000 mg per day

NUTRITIONAL APPROACHES

Eat daily helpings of kale, broccoli, Brussels sprouts, bitter greens, cabbage, bok choy, and radishes, and get plenty of fiber in your diet. Carrots and sweet potatoes are rich sources of beta-carotene, which may help reduce a wide range of cancers like lung, mouth, throat, and breast cancer. Avocadoes are a wonderful source of glutathione—the liver's most important antioxidant. Make sure you're eating at least 4 oz/115 g of protein per meal and 2 oz/55 g at each snack to help the liver make glutathione. Incorporate fresh herbs and spices like garlic, cilantro, and chili peppers, which may neutralize cancer-causing substances, into your recipes.

Digestive Woes

This protocol relieves abdominal bloating from gas, constipation, food sensitivities, and low levels of digestive enzymes.

SUPPLEMENTS

Magnesium	400 mg twice per day on an empty stomach
Probiotics	8 to 16 billion organisms per day
Betaine hydrochloride	200 mg per meal (steer clear if you have a history of ulcers)

To optimize your digestion, aim for 9 to 12 daily servings of leafy green vegetables, and make sure at least 8 of those servings are derived from raw veggies. Raw vegetables are rich in digestive enzymes and fiber and will naturally slough off old bacteria from your intestinal walls, facilitating regular bowel movements. You can also make one meal per day purely vegetables and 1 cup/225 g of legumes like lentils or kidney beans for a fiber-reach meal. Steer clear of milk and cheese, which can be constipating, but incorporate plain yogurt or kefir for probiotic benefits. And make sure you sprinkle 2 tbsp ground flaxseeds on your oats or salads for an additional 6 g fiber per day. Stay hydrated with 8 to 12 glasses of water per day to help the fiber move through your system. Here's to smooth moves!

Energy

No one ever says they want less energy as they age! The secret to looking great is feeling great, which is as close as your next meal. Eat your protein first at meals and drop sugar out of your diet. Whole foods will optimize your energy levels and help you bid adieu to unwanted pounds and bloating. Keep your caffeine intake minimal so you don't blow out your adrenal glands. And don't forget to exercise, because energy begets energy!

PRE-WORKOUT: ENERGIZER BUNNY MOCKTAIL

If you work out first thing in the morning or just feel sluggish before your workouts, give this protocol a whirl for one month. You should notice an improvement in your energy and endurance. You'll probably notice that you're able to milk out a few more reps in your weight lifting sets and add heavier weights during your workouts. Have fun!

L-carnitine	2,000 mg per day
Rhodiola rosea	100 mg per day, taken first thing in the morning
BCAAs	20 g per day
CoQ10	300 mg per day
Lipoic acid	300 mg per day

Fat Loss

The following protocol will put your body in prime position to burn fat. These nutrients work synergistically with each other to facilitate your body's fat-burning mechanisms:

SUPPLEMENTS

CoQ10	200 mg per day
L-carnitine	2 to 5 g, two or three times per day
Omega-3s	1 tbsp fish oil twice per day for 6 months
GLA or primrose oil	2 capsules per day
Vitamin D_3	10,000 IU every other day until your blood test shows your levels at 80 to 120 ng/dL
Organic coconut oil	1 tbsp per day

NUTRITIONAL APPROACHES

Drink green tea as your caffeine source for best fat-loss results. If you must drink coffee, drink it within the hour before or after your workouts. Eat every 3 to 4 hours to rev up your metabolic rate and eat a serving of whole-food carbohydrates at night to balance your post-workout cortisol!

Muscle Relief

Please reference pages 59–60 for a full review on magnesium and its benefits.

POST-WORKOUT MUSCLE MOCKTAIL

This potent combination of nutrients will relieve sore muscles if you take it immediately following a workout:

1. 10–20 g BCAAs
2. 400 mg magnesium glycinate
3. 200 mg CoQ10
4. ½ tsp topical magnesium behind the knees
5. Repletion protein shake: 1 tbsp L-glutamine powder, 2 scoops whey or pea protein, 1 cup berries, 1 scoop greens powder, 1 cup water, cinnamon, stevia to sweeten. Blend with ice. If you're not feeling it with

a shake, have a meal of 4 scrambled egg whites with a side of ¼ cup/55 g dry oat bran mixed with 1 tsp cinnamon and ½ cup/120 mL water (boiled for 5 minutes), and 1 orange.

Sleep Restoration

Having recovered from debilitating insomnia, which I suffered through for years after my son was born, I can speak quite authentically on the subject of sleep. Sleep recovery is complex because the root cause can be multifactorial. There are a few different approaches you can take for sleep that will cover all the bases:

EXERCISE-INDUCED INSOMNIA

If you are overtraining and waking up at three in the morning, you need to lower your level of cortisol with the following nutrients. Take them with dinner or 2 hours before bed:

Phosphatidylserine	300 to 800 mg
Vitamin C ester	1,000 to 3,000 mg
Vitamin B$_6$	50 mg

Incorporate 10 minutes of meditation at bedtime; deep breathing is remarkably effective at lowering cortisol. One of my favorite meditation CDs is *A Meditation to Help You with Healthful Sleep* by Belleruth Naparstek, available at www.healthjourneys.com. Also, eat 2 oz/55 g of turkey breast an hour before bedtime to offset low blood sugar and boost serotonin levels in the brain.

ANXIETY-INDUCED INSOMNIA

If your wheels are spinning and you can't quiet your mind, try the following strategies:

- Cognitive behavioral therapy is an essential part of addressing anxiety and rewiring the brain; it helps to break the vicious cycle of repetitive thoughts and behaviors. Meditation is also a helpful activity (see CD mentioned above).
- Drink Yogi Bedtime Tea throughout the day if your anxiety is severe, and steep up to 3 bags at one time; otherwise drink 1 cup/240 ml with dinner or before bed while soaking in an Epsom salts bath.

- Try taking the following combination of nutrients when anxiety strikes throughout the day or an hour before bedtime:

Inositol	1 tsp in powder up to 3 times per day
CatecholeCalm	3 capsules up to 2 times per day (www.designsforhealth.com)
Magnesium glycinate	400 mg up to 3 times per day
5-HTP	200 mg per day
Taurine	2,000 mg per day

- Have a small piece of fruit with five almonds before bed to boost serotonin levels.

Sugar Cravings

Sugar cravings are often the result of missing nutrients and/or inadequate protein. Taking the following nutrients together will help stabilize your blood sugar and blast your cravings into oblivion.

SUPPLEMENTS

Lipoic acid	300 mg per day
L-glutamine	1 tbsp/5,000 mg per day in water or juice
Whey or pea protein	1 scoop (in a smoothie or water)
Magnesium glycinate	400 mg per day
5-HTP	200 mg per day
Rhodiola rosea	100 mg per day; best taken first thing in the morning

NUTRITIONAL APPROACHES

The sugar cravings protocol works great for weight loss, smoking cessation, and general cravings. It is essential to eat enough protein and fiber throughout the day to sustain your blood sugar and kick those cravings to the curb. It's also helpful to have 1 tbsp cocoa powder dissolved in hot water daily to boost serotonin and dopamine levels in the brain and help you relax. Bliss!

Get Hip to Immune Support

Got kids in school? Then you probably need to give them immune support, too! Elderberry syrup tastes delish and may help fend off H1N1 virus. Give 1 tsp twice daily for prevention, and 2 tsp four times daily with an active cold. Sambucol makes a good product, but you can also make your own. Here's to Gorgeous Health this winter!

ELDERBERRY SYRUP

In a large saucepan, cover 2 oz/55 g dried elderberries with 4 cups/960 ml water. Bring to a boil. Lower the heat and simmer over low heat until reduced to 2 cups/480 ml. Remove from the heat and strain. Add 1 1/2 cups/510 g honey to the liquid and stir until dissolved. Cool to room temperature and pour into a clean jar with a tight-fitting lid. Label with the date; syrup will keep up to 1 year in the refrigerator.

Vitamin D Deficiency

See page 58 for information on the importance of vitamin D in the body.

SUPPLEMENTS

Vitamin D_3	10,000 IU every other day for 3 months (www.designsforhealth.com); then have your levels retested.
Vitamin K_1	500 mcg per day
Vitamin K_2	500 mcg per day
Vitamin A	5,000 IU per day

She says: A couple of months ago, I had a bout of either stomach flu or food poisoning. After a day of nausea, diarrhea, and consuming only liquids to stay hydrated, I awoke the next morning feeling amazing. In fact, I felt so good that I began to wonder if the virus or food poisoning wasn't actually good for me. I've heard people talk about colon cleansing and I'm wondering if this is what all the hype is about. Are products that promise colon cleansing or detoxification safe? Can these aid weight loss? (Like everyone else, I'd like to lose that bit of fat congregating around my midsection.) How often should one "cleanse" the colon? Finally, would this interfere with my daily exercise? (I'm assuming it would.)

E says: I'm guessing you felt amazing because you were no longer vomiting or having diarrhea, but it could also have been due to the fasting component of it all. Usually, when people feel better after fasting, it means they have some food sensitivities. Removing the offending substances (like gluten or dairy, for example) gives the gut a much-needed break. Prolonged exposure to food allergens can cause leaky gut syndrome, which causes the gut to become semipermeable, allowing large, undigested particles to pass back and forth between the intestinal wall and the peritoneal cavity. That would make anyone feel tired, bloated, and sluggish!

Colon cleanses are usually safe, but I don't recommend them because I think they're just a waste of money. Detoxification should occur on a daily basis; it's impossible for the body to eliminate years of toxic exposure in only a few days. Colon cleanses probably clean up some residual constipation and digestive issues that plague so many people, and it's a good quick fix for those problems. But on a long-term basis you can keep your colon squeaky clean by eating enough fiber through fruits, vegetables, fresh green juices, ground flaxseeds, and fiber powders; eating adequate protein on a daily basis; drinking plenty of water to flush the colon; and enjoying hypoallergenic starches like sweet potatoes, brown rice, winter squashes, and root vegetables. All of these foods promote an alkaline environment and optimal digestion—and, ultimately, weight loss, too. (For specific meal plan suggestions, including gluten-free options, see pages 100–125.)

To lose the weight you mentioned, make sure you are only doing intense cardio intervals (instead of long cardio sessions) and lifting heavy weights at the gym, and walking on your "rest days." This will restore hormonal balance in your body and decrease the hormone cortisol, which can often contribute to weight stored around your midsection. Good luck!

She says: I am a vegan and constantly worried about getting enough vitamins and protein in my diet. My hair is dry and my nails tend to split—a lot! I used to have very tough nails but now they split weekly. What vegan supplements can you recommend for splitting nails and dry hair?

E says: Sounds to me like you need an oil change and a protein boost! Food first: Incorporate protein into your diet by supplementing with shakes. Designs for Health makes a pea- and rice-based protein powder (Paleomeal DF) that you can blend with almond milk, fresh fruit, flaxseeds, and ice. Make yourself two shakes per day (4 scoops total). Also, consume 5 g of BCAAs mixed into water twice per day to preserve lean muscle mass. To combat dry hair, you will need to take 2 tbsp per day of Udo's 3-6-9 Oil Blend, which contains a balanced combination of omega-3, -6, and -9—great for hydrating and lubricating your rockin' bod from the inside out! Last, steer completely clear of hydrogenated oils and fried foods— they will literally pull the good fats out of your body and displace them with unhealthy, pro-inflammatory fats that will leave you dry as the Sahara. You'll also need to take 500 mg calcium, 400 mg magnesium glycinate, 5,000 IU vitamin D_3, and a good trace mineral formulation daily.

She says: Are all supplements FDA approved? Should I take a day off once a week when taking herbs or supplements?

E says: Nope, supplements are not FDA approved—not one iota. But this isn't a bad thing; it just means you should work with a nutritionist or a nutritionally oriented physician to determine what supplements are right for you. You can take a day off from supplements, if you wish—sometimes our busy schedules just get the best of us and we forget, anyway. But if you are on a prescribed regimen to treat a specific condition, run it by your practitioner first. Often you will need to take them every day to get the best results. I personally find that my energy dips tremendously if I don't take my multivitamin and adrenal support, leading to cravings and dragginess. As a result, I prefer to take them every day.

She says: What are the best supplements for an individual to take while preparing for a triathlon? Are protein-rich meal replacement bars and drinks the way to go? How much protein is too much? Is it better to eat real foods rather than recovery-type substances?

E says: I'm so glad you asked! Due to their heavy cardio component, triathlons are catabolic to the body, so protein is your number-one priority. Make sure that you are eating at least 0.035 to 0.042 oz/1 to 1.2 g of protein per 1 lb/0.5 kg of body weight, in order to fight muscle wasting during training. Pair this at each meal with recovery-friendly complex carbs, such as sweet potatoes, brown rice, legumes, hummus, and winter squashes. If your workouts are longer than an hour, you will need to ingest either a commercial power gel (I like CarbBoom Gel, which has a fruit-puree base) or make your own (see page 98). Consume one juice or gel per hour of your long workout, with plenty of water in between. Protein bars and smoothies are a quick and easy way to make sure you're getting enough protein. On page 97, I've also included a Gatorade substitute, which works beautifully for the longer workouts. Both pre- and post-workout, make sure you take BCAAs (10 g) in your water to nourish your muscles and prevent wasting. And on your "off days," make sure you walk to flush lactic acid and stiffness from your legs and lower your cortisol levels.

Finally, take the following nutrients with breakfast to replace glycogen stores and boost energy:

CoQ10	200 mg
Alpha-lipoic acid	400 mg
L-carnitine	2,000 to 4,000 mg
Omega-3s	1 tbsp liquid per day
BioDrive	2 capsules per day (from Biotics Research; contains rhodiola rosea for adrenal support)

During and after an endurance event, repletion of fluids, electrolytes, and carbohydrates is critical. Quite often, the commercial synthetic sports drinks and power gels are very high in sugar, which can irritate the stomach and lead to bloating and cramping. On pages 97–98 are two recipes that are easy to digest and can help optimize your performance and recovery. They take only a little extra effort to put together and can mean the difference between feeling good and feeling great.

GORGEOUS
IN THE KITCHEN

E very woman should have at least five main courses she can cook well. I've included staples from my personal repertoire that you can make quickly and easily. Although I'm a competent cook and am not afraid to make mistakes, I like to keep it simple for weeknights, when I don't have a lot of time, and save the more elaborate cooking for the weekends. Try these for yourself and see if they don't become a regular part of your repertoire as well!

You'll notice that most of these recipes serve four to six people. If you don't need to feed this many people, you can either cut the recipe in half or make the whole thing and eat or freeze the leftovers. The main courses freeze well, but the vegetables should probably just be eaten for lunch or dinner the next day. The benefit of having leftovers is that you save a ton of cash during the course of the week and you're doing your body justice by eating healthfully all the while. Also, note that the recipes are basically gluten free, so everyone can get a piece of the action. Not too shabby!

To up the ante, see page 99 for some excellent substitutes that will improve the nutritional value of what you are eating without compromising the taste.

Roasted Chicken

Roasting chicken is as easy as 1-2-3! Preheat the oven to 350°F/180°C. Chop up onions, garlic, bell peppers, mushrooms, and potatoes. Toss with fresh parsley, sea salt, pepper, and 2 tbsp olive oil. Transfer the vegetables to a roasting pan and spread evenly. Top with a whole chicken (approximately 10 lb/4.5 kg) rubbed with melted butter, salt, and pepper, and stuffed with a few sprigs of fresh thyme. Roast for 1 hour, or until the juices run clear. When the chicken seems cooked, insert an instant-read thermometer into the breast. It should read 180°F/82°C. Let the chicken rest 5 minutes before serving.

The Healthiest Eggs

The best way to cook eggs is using the method I call "low and slow." The chemical bonds of protein in eggs are extremely delicate and can be damaged at high temperatures (the same goes for the fat you are cooking with). So, instead of frying your eggs, turn your burner on low to medium heat and add 1 tsp olive oil to your skillet. Add your eggs or egg whites and allow them to cook slowly over low heat for a few minutes. Feel free to add vegetable toppings like sautéed onions, asparagus, mushrooms, tomatoes, and spinach to beef up the antioxidant content. Serve atop high-fiber, high-protein hemp toast with a side of organic berries. Breakfast is served!

Winter Frittata

Tired of the same ol' beef, chicken, or fish for dinner? Try this amazingly healthful and satisfying frittata. It's packed with protein and veggies, so you can't go wrong! Of course, it works great for brunch, too.

SERVES 6

5 slices turkey bacon (look for nitrate-free, lean-cut versions)

2 large red potatoes, thinly sliced

2 medium red onions, sliced

½ red bell pepper, chopped

2 tsp dried rosemary

½ tsp sea salt

2 tbsp olive oil

2 cups/60 g chopped spinach

1 garlic clove, minced

4 whole eggs

8 egg whites

½ tsp black pepper

4 oz/115 g reduced-fat feta, crumbled, or 4 oz/115 g shredded almond cheese

In a 10-in/25-cm skillet, cook the bacon until crisp. Remove from the pan, let cool, chop, and set aside. In the same pan, sauté the potatoes, onions, bell pepper, rosemary, and ¼ tsp of the salt in 1 tbsp of the olive oil for 5 minutes over medium heat. Cover and cook 10 minutes more. Stir in the spinach and garlic and sauté for 1 minute. Remove from the heat. Beat the eggs, egg whites, and remaining ¼ tsp salt in a large bowl. Add the vegetables, bacon, black pepper, and cheese. Preheat the broiler, and wipe the skillet clean. Place the skillet over medium heat and add the remaining 1 tbsp olive oil, ensuring that it evenly covers the base and sides of the pan. Pour in the egg mixture and cook for 4 minutes. Move the skillet to the broiler and broil, uncovered, for 3 minutes. Slide the frittata onto a plate, cut into six wedges, and serve hot or cool.

Chicken with Lemon-Basil Sauce

I love to cook this in the dead of winter because its light, lemony flavor reminds me of a lovely vacation spent in Positano. Pair it with some sautéed spinach and transport yourself to la dolce vita!

SERVES 4

3 tbsp grapeseed oil
4 organic skinless boneless chicken breast halves (sliced in half if large)
Salt and pepper
3 tbsp lemon juice from organic lemons
1 packed tsp grated lemon peel
4 garlic cloves, chopped
1 cup/240 ml low-salt chicken broth
⅓ cup/70 g chopped fresh basil

In a heavy 10-in/25-cm skillet, heat the grapeseed oil over medium-high heat. Meanwhile, sprinkle the chicken with salt and pepper. Add the chicken to the skillet and sauté until brown and cooked through, about 5 minutes per side. Transfer the chicken to a platter and tent with foil. Add the lemon juice, lemon peel, and garlic to the skillet. Stirring constantly, cook over medium-high heat until fragrant, about 30 seconds. Add the chicken broth to the skillet and bring to a boil until the mixture thickens, about 8 minutes. Stir in the basil and season with salt and pepper. Spoon the sauce over the chicken and serve.

Gorgeous Eating 101

Eating clean involves more than just choosing healthful food; it also means cleaning your food before you eat it! Of the "clean foods" we eat, 90 percent of them are wrapped in plastic, so rinse everything before you eat it to remove any plastic residue. I believe safe food storage is just as important as the food we're eating, due to plastic's potential for hormonal disruption. Glass containers with snap-on lids are the safest bet and will help reduce your exposure to toxins.

Turkey Meatballs

This recipe is a weekly staple in my home. To mix it up, I sometimes use ground grass-fed beef or buffalo in place of ground turkey. Do as you see fit! You can also incorporate different spices to please your palate. For best results, make the meatballs up to a day in advance so the flavors get sealed in. They freeze well, too. When buying tomato sauce, look for a high-quality, sugar-free sauce in a jar. It really makes a difference! Feel free to make your own sauce, too.

SERVES 4 TO 6

1 lb/455 g ground turkey

¼ cup/20 g ground whole rolled oats (use rice flour or pulverized rice crackers for gluten-free options)

1 garlic clove, crushed

1 tsp onion powder

4 tbsp/15 g chopped fresh parsley or 2 tbsp dried parsley

Dash each of oregano, basil, salt, and pepper

1 tbsp plus 1 tsp grapeseed oil

24-oz/680-g jar organic tomato sauce

Combine the turkey, oats, garlic, onion powder, parsley, oregano, basil, salt, and pepper in a medium-size bowl and shape into 1½-in-/3.5-cm-diameter meatballs. Add the grapeseed oil to a 10-in/25-cm skillet and place over low heat. When the oil is warm, add the meatballs and brown them on all sides over low to medium heat. Add the tomato sauce, evenly coating the meatballs. Cover and simmer for 30 minutes. Remove from the heat and serve.

Buffalo Meatloaf with Spinach and Roasted Baby Potatoes

This is a complete meal with a main course and two sides. Buffalo tastes slightly sweeter than beef and has significantly less fat. You can find buffalo at upscale grocery stores and specialty food stores, some farmers' markets, and online. You can also use grass-fed beef or ground turkey in this recipe. When using ground oats for this and other recipes, you will need to grind whole oats by running them through a coffee grinder for 10 seconds, or until they are pulverized into a powdery texture.

SERVES 4 TO 6

1 lb/455 g baby Yukon gold or Dutch yellow potatoes
⅓ cup/75 ml olive oil
6 oz/170 g mushrooms, chopped
1 medium red onion, chopped
1 tbsp chopped fresh sage
1 tbsp chopped fresh thyme
1 lb/455 g ground buffalo meat
1 large egg
¾ cup/190 g tomato sauce
½ cup/80 g ground rolled oats (rice flour or pulverized rice crackers for
  gluten-free options)
Sea salt
½ tsp cracked black pepper
1 garlic clove, pressed
10-oz/280-g bag fresh spinach

Preheat the oven to 375°F/190°C. In a medium bowl, toss the potatoes with 1 tbsp of the olive oil. Place the potatoes in a 13-by-9-in/33-by-23-cm glass pan or roasting pan. Roast in the oven for 45 minutes. Remove from the oven and set aside.

Meanwhile, heat 2 tbsp of the olive oil in a medium skillet over medium heat. Add the mushrooms and onion; sauté until mushrooms are beginning to brown and the onion is translucent, about 4 minutes. Remove from the heat and stir in the sage and thyme. Let cool slightly.

Mix together the buffalo meat, mushroom mixture, egg, ½ cup/125 g of the tomato sauce, oats, salt, and pepper in large bowl. Push the potatoes to the sides of the baking pan; shape the buffalo mixture into a 6-by-3-in/15-by-7.5-cm loaf in center of sheet. Roast for 30 minutes. Pour the remaining ¼ cup/60 g tomato sauce over the top of the meatloaf and roast for 20 minutes longer. Remove from the oven; let rest while preparing the spinach.

Heat the remaining 2 tbsp olive oil and the garlic in large pot over medium-high heat. Add spinach and toss until wilted, about 3 minutes. Slice the meatloaf and serve potatoes and spinach alongside.

Simple Salmon

Wild Alaskan salmon is extremely versatile. Its slightly gamey flavor adds depth and texture to the toppings you pair it with. Try topping salmon with salsa and guacamole, olive oil and lemon, sundried tomatoes and roasted garlic, tomato sauce, fresh Parmesan, or pesto sauce. You can also grill it and slice it up over a bed of steamed spinach—simple perfection! Just remember to never overcook salmon, lest you be left with a dry and tasteless piece of pesce.

SERVES 4

Four 6-oz/170-g salmon fillet pieces
Olive oil

Preheat the oven to 400°F/200°C. Arrange the salmon pieces on a baking sheet or glass baking pan and lightly brush with olive oil. Roast for 6 minutes, or until fish is no longer translucent in the center. Serve immediately.

Veggies

McSteamy

Steaming is one of the easiest ways to prepare vegetables, and it can be done in minutes. You'll retain the vitamins in the vegetables while keeping their gorgeous color intact. Here's how to do it:

1. Cut, chop, and trim vegetables for steaming.
2. In a large pot, bring 2 in/5 cm of water to a boil over high heat.
3. Place the vegetables in the steamer or steamer basket and cover the pot with a tight-fitting lid.
4. Steam the vegetables only until tender; this usually takes about 2 to 3 minutes.
5. Drizzle with your favorite olive oil and a dash of sea salt. *Et voilà!* Crunchy and delish.

Grilled Vegetables

So many recipes recommend adding quite a lot of salt to grilled vegetables. I try to cook with little to no salt whenever possible and use onion powder instead. The flavor is so delicious that you won't miss the salt! Plus, you'll stay gorgeously bloat-free in your summer maillot. If you don't have a grill, feel free to roast the vegetables for 20 to 30 minutes at 400°F/200°C. Showcase your talents by artfully arranging the vegetables on a large platter.

SERVES 6

2 eggplants
2 summer squash
2 green zucchini
12 carrots, peeled
1 red onion
2 red, yellow, or orange bell peppers

4 garlic cloves, minced

1 cup grapeseed or coconut oil (these stand up well to high-heat temperatures)

1 tbsp onion powder

Slice the eggplants, squash, zucchini, and carrots into ½-in-/1-cm-thick slices. Slice the onion into thick discs that won't fall apart on the grill. Core, seed, and quarter the bell peppers. In a large bowl, combine the vegetables, garlic, oil, and onion powder. Toss to coat the vegetables in oil. Grill over a medium-hot fire for up to 45 minutes. Flip the vegetables a couple of times and cook until tender but not at all mushy or black. Serve immediately.

Salt and Vinegar Kale Chips

Kale is the new potato! These light and crunchy "chips" are practically guilt-free.

SERVES 8

2 bunches kale, rinsed with stems removed

1 tbsp apple cider vinegar

3 tbsp olive oil

1 tsp salt (or less, as desired)

Preheat the oven to 350°F/180°C. Line two baking sheets with parchment paper. Cut the kale into 2- to 3-in/5- to 7.5-cm pieces. In a large bowl, combine the vinegar, olive oil, and salt. Add the kale and toss by hand until all the leaves are covered. Evenly distribute the kale among the prepared baking sheets and bake for 20 minutes, or until the leaves are crispy. If the chips are not sizzling or crispy yet, turn up the heat to 400°F/200°C and bake for a few minutes more. Baking time varies depending on the size of your chips and desired crispness; note that the outer edges cook quicker than the pieces from near the stem. The chips are best if enjoyed immediately, but can keep overnight in an airtight container in the fridge.

Guacamole

This adaptation of Ina Garten's guacamole recipe is a hit every time I make it, and it complements fresh crudités, eggs, burgers, salmon, and chicken salad beautifully. We call guacamole "green butter" in our house because it can also replace butter or mayonnaise on bread. (Psst . . . Do you love avocadoes but have a hard time preventing the unused portion from turning brown? Try this amazing trick: Wrap them in aluminum foil before storing them in the fridge. It works!)

MAKES 3 CUPS

4 ripe Haas avocados
Freshly squeezed lemon juice from ½ lemon
4 dashes Tabasco sauce
1 small red onion, diced
1 large garlic clove, minced
Kosher salt
Freshly ground black pepper
1 medium tomato, seeded and diced

Cut the avocados in half lengthwise, remove the pits, and, with a large spoon, scoop the flesh out of their shells into a large bowl. Immediately add the lemon juice, Tabasco, onion, garlic, 1 tsp salt, and ½ tsp pepper. Using two large forks, mash the avocados in the bowl with the other ingredients until they reach your desired consistency. Stir in the tomato and season with salt and pepper before serving.

Gazpacho Tex-Mex Style

When you visit my folks in the heart of summer, you'll be hard pressed to find their fridge without a large container of this gazpacho inside. Quick and easy, it's the perfect appetizer for any summer meal. The beauty of this recipe is that you don't have to stand in front of a hot stove to make it!

46-oz/1.3-L can of tomato juice or V-8
Juice of 3 freshly squeezed lemons
1 medium green bell pepper, chopped
1 small onion, chopped
1 cucumber, peeled and chopped, plus additional for garnish
¼ tsp chili powder
2 dashes Tabasco sauce
1 tbsp Worcestershire sauce
2 garlic cloves
1 tbsp olive oil
1 tbsp chopped fresh chives
Kosher salt
Freshly ground black pepper
Fresh parsley, for garnish

Place all the ingredients in the blender (in batches if your blender won't hold all of the ingredients at once). Blend at slow speed until smooth or slightly chunky, depending on your preference. Chill well for several hours; taste and adjust seasonings as necessary. Serve with a garnish of additional chopped cucumbers and fresh parsley.

Simple Salad

This fresh, simple salad makes a wonderful appetizer for a hearty fall or winter dinner, when fennel and pomegranates are in season.

SERVES 4 TO 6

2 fennel bulbs

1 red onion

1 large grapefruit, peeled and sectioned

1 large orange, peeled and sectioned

1 cup/120 g fresh pomegranate seeds

1 tbsp olive oil

1 tsp freshly squeezed lemon juice

Wash and slice the fennel and onion into thin strips. Place in a large bowl with the citrus sections and pomegranate seeds. Gently toss with the olive oil and lemon juice. Serve at room temperature.

Tomato, Avocado, and Red Onion Salad

Another simple salad for you. Although the ingredients are inspired by gazpacho, this lush, refreshing salad complements the smoky flavors of grilled meats and vegetables.

SERVES 6

1 pt/455 g plum or Roma tomatoes, cut into wedges

1 small red onion, thinly sliced

½ cup/120 ml plus 2 tbsp extra virgin olive oil (and more for drizzling)

3 tbsp red wine vinegar

Fine sea salt

3 Haas avocadoes

Freshly ground black pepper

In a large bowl, combine the tomatoes, onion, olive oil, vinegar, and a big pinch of salt. Gently toss and divide among serving plates. Halve and pit the avocadoes; scoop out flesh with a large spoon and slice them facedown on a cutting board. Divide the avocadoes, arranging them on top of the tomato mixture. Sprinkle each plate with a small pinch of salt and pepper and drizzle with olive oil before serving.

Basic Brown Rice

Brown rice is the perfect balance between yin and yang. Easy to digest, hypoallergenic, and rich in B vitamins, this chewy grain is the go-to gal for a satisfying side dish.

SERVES 4

1 cup/190 g brown rice
2 cups/480 ml organic chicken stock (or vegetable broth for a vegetarian option)
½ cup/120 ml water
1 tsp onion powder
1 tbsp dried parsley
1 carrot, peeled and sliced

Combine the rice, stock, and water in a 2-qt/2-L saucepan over medium heat; cover. Bring to a boil; stir in the onion powder, parsley, and carrots and lower the heat. Simmer uncovered for 15 minutes, stirring occasionally, until all the liquid is absorbed or until the rice reaches the desired consistency. Serve immediately.

Polenta

Another simple yet delicious side dish that is low in calories and moderate in carbohydrate content. Polenta is incredibly versatile and can be topped with tomato sauce, meatballs, cheese, fresh tomatoes, or even guacamole and shredded chicken.

SERVES 4

16 oz/455 g tube premade organic polenta
Olive oil
Freshly grated Parmigiano Reggiano for garnish

Preheat the oven to 375°F/190°C. Line a metal baking sheet with aluminum foil. Remove the polenta from its plastic casing. Rinse well and pat dry. Cut the polenta log into even ¾-in/2-cm slices and place on the baking sheet. Lightly brush olive oil on both sides of the discs. Bake for 15 minutes and remove from the oven, turning the slices over with a spatula so they don't break apart. Grate fresh Parmigiano over the slices and place them back in the oven for another 15 minutes. Serve immediately.

Butternut Squash and Red Pepper Casserole

This recipe is the perfect header for fall, when root vegetables are at their peak. The fresh herbs really pop against the sweetness of the squash and pepper. Make sure you use a high-quality, organic olive oil packaged in a dark or opaque bottle for the freshest taste and highest nutritional value.

SERVES 6

One 3½ lb/1.6 kg butternut squash (look for pre-peeled and precut squash)
1 large red bell pepper, cut into 1-in/2.5-cm pieces
3 tbsp olive oil
2 large garlic cloves, minced
3 tbsp minced fresh parsley leaves
1½ tsp minced fresh rosemary leaves
Salt
Freshly ground black pepper
½ cup/50 g freshly grated Parmesan

Preheat the oven to 400°F/200°C. (If necessary, peel the whole squash, cut in half, and scoop out and discard seeds. With a sharp knife, cut squash into 1-in/2.5-cm cubes.) In a large bowl, toss the squash, bell pepper, olive oil, garlic, and herbs. Season with salt and pepper. Transfer the mixture to a 2-qt/2-L shallow baking dish and sprinkle evenly with the Parmesan. Bake until the squash is tender and the top is golden, about 1 hour. Serve immediately.

Sweet Potato "Fries"

I'm a simple gal and can eat baked sweet potatoes daily, but my family craves variety, so these baked fries are always a happy medium. The first time you make these, give them plenty of love and attention, as they can burn easily if you're not careful. Also bear in mind ovens always vary with cooking times, since very few ovens are perfectly calibrated!

2 tbsp coconut oil
4 sweet potatoes
Sea salt

Preheat the oven to 375°F/190°C. Line a metal baking sheet with aluminum foil and lightly brush with a little of the coconut oil. Wash and pat dry the sweet potatoes. Using a sharp knife, cut the sweet potatoes into fry-shaped slices about $\frac{1}{4}$ in/6 mm thick or to desired thickness (a thicker cut will prevent them from burning). Arrange the sweet potato slices on the baking sheet and brush the tops with the remaining coconut oil. Sprinkle very lightly with sea salt. Place in the oven, turning or flipping them every 5 minutes so they don't burn, until they reach desired crispness, about 25 minutes. Serve immediately.

Frankies Corn Salad

This recipe is slightly adapted from The Frankies Spuntino Kitchen Companion & Cooking Manual. *A summer hit for sure! To keep things simple, I like to substitute Trader Joe's frozen roasted corn in place of shucking and grilling fresh corn. But if the mood strikes you and you're feeling inspired, go for it with fresh grilled corn!*

SERVES 6

4 cups/655 g frozen roasted corn
1 pt/455 g cherry tomatoes, halved
2 tbsp torn mint leaves
½ medium red onion, sliced
3 tbsp olive oil
Juice of 1 lemon
Sea salt
Mild goat cheese (optional)

Gently defrost the corn in a skillet over medium heat until the kernels are evenly warmed. Transfer the corn to a big salad bowl. Add the tomatoes, and then the mint and onion, and toss. Drizzle with the olive oil and lemon juice and season with salt. Crumble goat cheese on top, if desired, before serving.

Sweet Treats

When I'm craving a sweet treat, I want the real deal. I always use sugar or honey in baking because it keeps me in check: I'm far more likely to eat less of the real deal than I would the fake stuff. However, there are a couple of pretty good sugar substitutes available, especially for those times when you want a treat but don't want to stray too far off track. These products are safe for diabetics, anyone who is insulin resistant or just wants to lose weight, and anyone who wants to lose body fat but still enjoy the taste of something sweet. So if you want some good old-fashioned chocolate chip cookies, indulge away. And if you want the version for the new millennium, then read on! Some of these recipes I've picked up from other bakers; they were simply too good not to pass on.

Coconut Flour Chocolate Cake

I love baking with coconut flour! It smells heavenly, and it's gluten-free and high in protein, which helps blunt the glycemic effect of sugar. I cut the sugar from the original recipe almost in half; you can also go completely sugar-free with xylitol, which can be found online or at health food stores. Good luck, and have fun!

SERVES 10

Coconut oil
1 cup/100 g unsweetened cocoa powder, plus additional for dusting pans
1 cup/225 g butter, at room temperature
1½ cup/300 g sugar (white or brown) or 1½ cup/285 g xylitol
10 eggs, at room temperature
½ tsp vanilla extract
2 cups/225 g coconut flour
1½ tsp baking soda
½ tsp baking powder
1 tsp salt
1⅓ cups/320 ml whole milk or almond milk
4 cups/910 g frosting of your choice

Preheat the oven to 350°F/180°C. Grease two 9-in/23-cm or 8-in/20-cm round layer pans with coconut oil and dust with cocoa powder. In a stand mixer fitted with the paddle attachment, beat the butter and sugar together for about 2 minutes. Add the eggs, one at a time, and beat at high speed for about 3 minutes; add the vanilla. In a separate bowl, combine the cocoa powder, coconut flour, baking soda, baking powder, and salt; add the flour mixture alternately with the milk to the butter mixture. Beat the batter for about 5 minutes more on high speed. Spoon the batter into the prepared cake pans and smooth out the tops.

Bake for 30 to 35 minutes, or until a toothpick inserted into the center of the cakes comes out clean. Place the pans on wire racks and let cool for 10 minutes before removing from the pans. Let the cakes cool completely before using your favorite frosting to frost the cake.

Gluten-Free and Vegan Chocolate Chip Cookies

Almond flour is another great gluten-free option for baking, and you can either purchase it or make it yourself in a food processor. To make it yourself, dump blanched almonds in a food processor and pulse until they turn to almond meal. Don't overdo it, though, or you'll end up with almond butter instead!

MAKES 24 COOKIES

2½ cups/280 g Trader Joe's almond flour
½ tsp baking soda
½ tsp Celtic sea salt
½ cup/120 ml grapeseed oil
½ cup/170 g honey or agave nectar
1 tbsp vanilla extract
1 cup/170 g dark chocolate chips (look for chocolate chips with 73 percent cacao)

Preheat the oven to 350°F/180°C. Line a baking sheet with parchment. In a large bowl, combine the almond flour, baking soda, and salt. In a medium bowl, combine the grapeseed oil, honey, and vanilla, stirring until blended. Add the oil-and-honey mixture to the flour mixture and stir until combined. Stir in the chocolate chips. Form 1-in/2.5-cm balls and press onto the parchment-lined baking sheet. Bake the cookies for 7 to 10 minutes, or until lightly browned. Let the cookies cool before serving.

Low-Carb Chocolate Peanut Butter Bars

This recipe was masterminded by amazing fitness and strength coach Jill Coleman.
Jill walks the walk when it comes to eating clean and exercising. She loves to cook
and create moderate indulgences so she can have her cake and eat it, too. These bars are
lower in carbs but still high in fat and calories, so keep your portion size to one bar only!

MAKES 24 BARS

1 cup/225 g unsalted butter
2 cups/8 oz pecan flour (or pecans ground in the food processor)
1¾ cup Ideal Confectioner's sugar
1¼ cups/325 g natural peanut butter
4 oz/115 g baking chocolate (look for at least 70 percent cacao)
1 tbsp xylitol or erythritol

In a large bowl, beat together the butter, pecan flour, and confectioner's sugar.
Add 1 cup/260 g of the peanut butter and beat well. Spread the mixture in an
ungreased 9-by-13-in/23-by-33-cm pan. In a small saucepan, melt the chocolate
with the remaining ¼ cup/65 g peanut butter over low heat, stirring until combined
and melted. Remove from the heat and add the xylitol to sweeten. Pour the chocolate mixture over the peanut butter mixture in the baking pan until it evenly covers
the whole batch with a thin layer of chocolate. Cover and place the pan in the fridge
for at least 1 hour until firm. Cut into bars and enjoy!

Sweet Dreams

Xylitol and erythritol can be used in any recipe that calls for sugar. Both are
sugar alcohols, and both are very low on the glycemic index (xylitol has a GI of
seven; erythritol has a GI of zero). The only downside is that xylitol is a prebiotic
that can rank pretty high on the fart scale—but it usually becomes better
tolerated with continued use. When used in baking, erythritol and xylitol don't
caramelize, so you'll need to add more liquid to retain moisture.

Protein Smoothie

This protein smoothie is an incredibly useful tool for weight loss and appetite control. Experiment with variations—you won't be disappointed. Bon appétit, my sweet!

1 scoop whey powder, pea, or rice protein
1 heaping tbsp ground flaxseeds
1 cup/150 g fresh or frozen blueberries
1 cup/240 ml almond milk or water
1 tbsp unsweetened cocoa powder
Ice
Cinnamon for garnish

In a blender, combine the protein powder, flaxseeds, blueberries, almond milk, and cocoa powder and 5 ice cubes (for an extra-slushy treat, add 2 cups of ice) and blend on high speed. Sprinkle with cinnamon before serving.

Sports Repletion Drink

For the high-octane junkies out there training for marathons, triathlons, and Iron Man competitions, stay nourished and hydrated with the following homemade remedies on the days you do your long workouts.

1 cup/240 ml organic juice, such as apple or grape
1 cup/240 ml water
⅓ tsp sea salt
1,000 mg L-carnitine, in powdered form

Combine all ingredients in a sealable bottle and shake well. Store for up to 24 hours in the refrigerator.

Homemade Power Gel

2 tbsp raw organic honey
2 tbsp raw peanut butter, 2 tbsp apple butter, or ½ banana
1 tsp lemon juice (to cut the sweetness)

In a blender, combine the honey and peanut butter until smooth and creamy. Add the lemon juice and blend again. Transfer to a fuel belt bottle and carry during a long run.

Butter

Butter up, buttercup! Contrary to popular opinion, butter is natural, safe, and healthy for you to eat. Our bodies need saturated fats to support our bones, protect the liver from toxins, enhance the immune system, and absorb omega-3s. Saturated fats also protect the heart muscle. And, only 26 percent of the fat in artery clogs is saturated; the rest is unsaturated. So enjoy your buttah—I love mine on broccoli! (This recipe is from Blue Hill at Stone Barns.)

MAKES 2 CUPS

5 cups/1.2 L heavy cream
Coarse salt

Using the whisk attachment of a stand mixer, beat the heavy cream at high speed until it achieves the consistency of whipped cream. Continue to beat the cream, scraping down the sides of the bowl occasionally with a rubber spatula. The cream will slowly begin to turn a light yellow color and take on a slightly granular appearance. When you start to see a watery liquid separate from the mass of yellowish butter solids, stop the mixer. Transfer the mixture to a fine-mesh sieve set over a bowl and start to squeeze as much liquid as possible from the mass of butter by gently pressing it against the sieve. Transfer the butter to a bowl and season lightly with coarse salt. Store in an airtight glass container in the fridge, or freeze until ready to use.

Sexy Substitutes

Boost the nutritional content of your recipes with the following substitutions that are nutritious and delicious!

IF YOU'RE USING . . .	TRY . . .
Breadcrumbs	Ground rolled oats (grind finely in coffee grinder)
Butter	Grapeseed or coconut oil
Corn syrup	Honey, agave, xylitol, or erythritol
Dried herbs (1 tsp)	Fresh herbs (1 tbsp)
Ketchup (1 cup)	1 cup/250 g tomato sauce + 2 tbsp vinegar + 1 packet stevia
Mayonnaise	Yogurt
Milk	Almond milk
Oil in baking (1 cup)	½ cup/120 g unsweetened applesauce + ½ cup/120 oil
Pasta	Pasta made from organic whole wheat with omega-3, 100 percent soba, quinoa, rice, or *shirataki*
Peanut butter, commercial	Peanut or almond butter, natural
Sifted white flour (1 cup)	1 cup/160 g ground rolled oats or coconut flour + 2½ tsp baking powder
White sugar (1 cup)	¾ cup/255 g honey; subtract ¼ cup/60 ml liquid from rest of recipe Or ¾ cup/255 g honey + ¼ cup/30 g flour + ¼ tsp baking soda; lower the oven temp 25°F/4°C Or 1 cup/190 g xylitol or agave (use ⅔ cup/125 g for baking; ½ cup/95 g in regular cooking)

MEAL PLANS

I have concocted four different meal plans to get you started. Choose the one that feels right for you. You may need to adjust the portion sizes or substitute other options if you don't care for the choices I've listed. Give yourself some time to get on track; it will be smooth sailing once you do.

No matter which meal plan you choose to follow, what you drink throughout the day will have a big impact on your health and how you feel. I highly recommend drinking water, sparkling water, club soda, herbal teas (peppermint, licorice, ginger, chamomile, raspberry, pomegranate, cinnamon, apple), or green tea (limit to 8 oz/240 ml per day). For a good coffee substitute, add 1 tbsp unsweetened cocoa powder to 10 oz/300 ml boiling water. Add a splash of milk and you have an antioxidant-rich bevvie!

Once per week, treat yourself to your favorite indulgence so you can keep your eye on the fitness prize while keeping your cravings in check. A brownie or cookie, ½ cup/120 mL of ice cream, or half of a chocolate bar can really satisfy the soul. If you need a little something sweet every night, try a couple squares of 70-percent-cacao dark or sugar-free chocolate. It will keep your taste buds humming and your fitness goals on track! Have fun, and feel gorgeous!

Low Carb and Loving It!

If you can't shake that muffin top and your pants are somewhat snug after a pasta meal, then it's time to switch out processed carbs for smaller amounts of more complex starches from fruits and vegetables. Following this plan for 4 weeks, along with exercise 4 days per week, can help you lose 8 to 10 lb/3.6 to 4.5 kg of water and body fat. Stay on this plan until you've reached your goal weight. Then you can add in one to two portions per day of fiber-rich starches, like brown rice, slow-cooked oats, sweet potatoes, winter squash, or beans and legumes. If you find you are hungry on this plan, add more protein, make sure you drink plenty of water, and increase your fiber by eating unlimited amounts of vegetables. You should find that your energy soars and your cravings disappear after 5 to 7 days.

DAY 1

Breakfast: 3 scrambled eggs cooked in 1 tsp butter, 1 cup/150 g berries sprinkled with 1 tbsp crushed pecans

Snack: 1 apple sliced and smeared with 1 tbsp almond butter

Lunch: 5 oz/140 g turkey burger over a spinach salad with ½ avocado, a slice of tomato, and red onions

Snack: ¼ cup/30 g raw nuts and 1 orange

Dinner: 6-oz/185-g can of chicken mixed with 1 tbsp raw apple cider and 2 tsp mayonnaise. Serve inside a raw bell pepper with ¼ avocado and carrot sticks on the side.

DAY 2   **Breakfast:** Omelet: 3 scrambled eggs, 1 chopped tomato, ¼ onion cooked in 1 tsp olive oil; 1 cup/150 g fresh blueberries

Snack: ¼ cup/30 g mixed raw nuts

Lunch: Crabmeat salad made with a 6-oz/170-g can of crabmeat, 1 chopped celery rib, 1 chopped scallion. Dress with ¼ cup/55 g yogurt and juice of ½ lemon, and serve inside ½ avocado. 1 cup/165 g strawberries. (Extra credit: buy organic fresh or frozen strawberries.)

Snack: 2 oz/55 g turkey jerky, 1 orange bell pepper

Dinner: 6 oz/170 g grilled chicken, sliced yellow squash and zucchini sautéed with ½ cup/120 ml chicken broth and 1 clove crushed garlic

DAY 3   **Breakfast:** Protein Smoothie (page 97)

Snack: 1 sliced orange and 1 hard-boiled egg

Lunch: 12 grilled shrimp atop Caesar salad; skip the croutons

Snack: 1 sliced bell pepper and ½ cup/120 g guacamole

Dinner: 5 Turkey Meatballs (page 83), 1 cup/180 g sautéed spinach, 8 asparagus spears

DAY 4   **Breakfast:** 2 turkey sausages, 1 sliced tomato, ¼ avocado

Snack: 2 celery ribs smeared with 2 tbsp almond butter

Lunch: Large salad with 5 olives, 1 tomato, ½ orange bell pepper, ½ cucumber, 1 celery stalk. Add a 6-oz/170-g can of chicken. (Extra credit: Have sardines, octopus, tuna, or salmon.) Drizzle with 2 tsp olive oil and fresh lemon juice.

Snack: 2 oz/55 g turkey jerky, handful of cherry tomatoes

Dinner: 6 oz/170 g buffalo burger (or substitute turkey) with roasted asparagus. (Wash 1 bunch of asparagus and place on a baking sheet. Drizzle with 2 tsp olive oil. Bake for 15 minutes at 350°F/180°C. Sprinkle fresh Parmesan atop spears and serve.)

DAY 5   **Breakfast:** 4 oz/110 g canned wild Alaskan salmon mixed with 1 tsp mayo and 1 tsp apple cider vinegar, 2-in/5-cm cantaloupe wedge. (If you can't stomach salmon for breakfast, try 2 turkey sausages with ½ cup/115 g cooked oats or a Protein Smoothie, page 97.)

Snack: ¼ cup/30 g mixed raw nuts

Lunch: Beef carpaccio salad topped with Parmesan and lemon, steamed artichokes

Snack: 2 oz/55 g sliced turkey breast rolled around ¼ avocado

Dinner: 6 oz/170 g grilled chicken, sliced yellow squash and zucchini sautéed with ½ cup/120 ml chicken broth and 1 clove crushed garlic

DAY 6   **Breakfast:** 1 cup/225 g Greek yogurt mixed with 1 scoop whey protein, ½ sliced banana, and 1 tbsp chopped walnuts

Snack: 1 cup/165 g sliced strawberries topped with 2 tbsp slivered almonds

Lunch: Roast beef wrap (4 oz/115 g roast beef wrapped in lettuce) with ½ avocado, side salad

Snack: 2 hard-boiled eggs and 10 almonds

Dinner: 6 oz/170 g Roasted Chicken (page 80), 1 cup/125 g steamed green beans (Steam until al dente and bright green; remove beans and place in bowl of ice water for 3 minutes to stop cooking and retain green color. Then place back in steamer to keep warm.)

DAY 7   **Breakfast:** 1 slice turkey bacon, 2 eggs, sunny-side up, cooked in 1 tsp butter, 1 cup/125 g raspberries. (Extra credit: Use organic berries.)

Snack: 2 celery ribs smeared with 2 tbsp natural peanut butter

Lunch: 5 oz/140 g grilled chicken salad with 1 tbsp each fresh dill, chopped red onion, garlic, and olive oil over 2 cups/60 g raw spinach, 1 apple

Snack: 1 cup/225 g plain yogurt with ½ cup/80 g sliced strawberries and 1 tbsp slivered almonds

Dinner: 6 oz/170 g filet mignon, 2 heads baby bok choy cooked in 1 tsp olive oil and sprinkled with sesame seeds

DAY 8

Breakfast: ½ cup/115 g cottage cheese topped with ½ cup/60 g raspberries, 2 slices of turkey bacon

Snack: ½ serving Protein Smoothie (page 97) or 1 banana with 1 tbsp peanut butter. (Extra credit: Use natural peanut butter)

Lunch: 5 oz/140 g buffalo burger (skip the bun) and a side salad with 1 tsp olive oil and 2 tsp vinegar

Snack: 2 oz/55 g sliced turkey breast rolled up around ¼ avocado

Dinner: 6 oz/170 g red snapper with ½ cup/80 g cooked wild rice and 1 cup/155 g roasted Brussels sprouts. (Wash and slice Brussels sprouts in half. Place in a medium bowl and toss with 2 tsp olive oil and a pinch of sea salt. Bake in a glass pan at 350°F/180°C for 45 minutes.)

DAY 9

Breakfast: 4 oz/110 g smoked salmon, ½ avocado, 2-in/5-cm cantaloupe wedge

Snack: ½ cup/115 g cottage cheese with ¼ cup/35 g blueberries

Lunch: Greek salad with 6 oz/170 g grilled chicken, drizzled with 2 tsp Italian dressing

Snack: 2 slices turkey breast rolled around ¼ avocado

Dinner: 5 oz/140 g lamb chop, sautéed broccoli rabe (1 bunch) sprinkled with sesame seeds. (Bake lamb chop for 15 to 20 minutes, depending on thickness, at 350°F/180°C on a baking sheet covered in foil or a glass or enamel pan.)

DAY 10

Breakfast: 2 slices Canadian bacon, ½ cup/115 g cottage cheese sprinkled with ½ cup/75 g blueberries

Snack: 1 apple sliced and smeared with 1 tbsp almond butter

Lunch: 1 cup/245 g turkey chili, 1 cup/155 g steamed broccoli, 1 pear

Snack: 1 cup/225 g plain yogurt with ½ cup/80 g sliced strawberries and 1 tbsp slivered almonds

Dinner: 6 oz/170 g lamb or chicken, cubed and skewered with red onions, bell peppers, and cherry tomatoes. Brush with olive oil and bake for 25 minutes at 350°F/180°C. Serve atop arugula salad topped with shaved Parmesan and 1 tsp pine nuts.

DAY 11   **Breakfast:** 4 oz/110 g smoked salmon, ¼ avocado, 1 sliced tomato, evenly distributed over 2 rye Wasa crackers, or Protein Smoothie (page 97)

Snack: ½ cup/115 g cottage cheese with ¼ cup/35 g blueberries

Lunch: 1 cup/245 g ginger-carrot soup (broth based), 4 oz/155 g beef carpaccio salad with lemon and Parmesan

Snack: 1 sliced orange and 2 hard-boiled eggs

Dinner: 6 oz/170 g chicken satay skewers, 3 vegetable dumplings, steamed vegetables

DAY 12   **Breakfast:** Protein Smoothie (page 97)

Snack: 1 cup/225 g plain yogurt with ½ cup/80 g sliced strawberries and 1 tbsp slivered almonds

Lunch: 6 oz/170 g chicken brushed with pesto or salsa, 1 cup/155 g roasted carrots

Snack: 1 apple sliced and smeared with 1 tbsp almond butter

Dinner: 6 oz/170 g wild Alaskan salmon (brush with 1 tsp pesto sauce, bake at 350°F/180°C for 7 to 8 minutes) with 1 cup/180 g sautéed spinach

DAY 13   **Breakfast:** 1 cup/225 g plain yogurt, ½ cup/85 g sliced strawberries, 1 tbsp ground flaxseeds, 1 tbsp chopped pecans. (Extra credit: Use organic yogurt.)

Snack: ¼ cup/30 g mixed raw nuts

Lunch: 5 oz/140 g turkey burger with 1 tbsp guacamole, red and yellow tomato salad drizzled with 1 tsp olive oil and fresh basil, 1 small ear corn on the cob

Snack: 1 sliced red bell pepper with ¼ cup/60 g hummus

Dinner: Omelet: 2 whole eggs plus 2 egg whites, ½ onion, and ½ red bell pepper. Serve with a side salad.

DAY 14

Breakfast: 3 scrambled eggs mixed with ¼ cup/40 g tomatoes and ¼ cup/40 g mushrooms, 1 cup/165 g sliced strawberries

Snack: 2 celery ribs and 2 tbsp natural peanut butter

Lunch: Beet and goat cheese salad with walnuts and 12 grilled shrimp

Snack: 2 oz/55 g sliced turkey breast, 5 almonds, 1 pear

Dinner: 6 oz/170 g buffalo burger with roasted asparagus. (Wash 1 bunch of asparagus and place on a baking sheet. Drizzle with 2 tsp olive oil. Bake for 15 minutes at 350°F/180°C. Sprinkle fresh Parmesan atop spears and serve.)

DAYS 15 TO 28: Repeat the cycle.

DAIRY- AND GLUTEN-FREE GIRL

Living gluten- and dairy-free can pose some challenges, but with a little creative energy you can make it work for you. Kinder living through clean eating will keep your tummy happy and give your body the tools it needs to absorb your nutrients. Clearing gluten from your diet can also help you drop stubborn body fat quickly and effectively. Gluten-free never looked more gorgeous!

DAY 1

Breakfast: Omelet: 3 scrambled eggs, 1 chopped tomato, ¼ onion cooked in 1 tsp olive oil; 1 cup/150 g fresh blueberries or any other fruit

Snack: 2 oz/55 g sliced turkey breast with mustard

Lunch: Large salad with 5 olives, 1 tomato, ½ orange bell pepper, ½ cucumber, 1 celery stalk. Add a 6-oz/170-g can of chicken. (Extra credit: Have sardines, octopus, tuna or salmon.) Drizzle with 2 tsp olive oil and fresh lemon juice. Apple slices for dessert.

Snack: 1 oz/30 g almond cheese with ½ cup/85 g sliced strawberries and 1 tbsp slivered almonds

Dinner: 6 oz/170 g grilled steak, sliced yellow squash and zucchini sautéed with chicken broth and garlic, ½ cup/100 g lentils sautéed with onions and cumin

DAY 2

Breakfast: Protein Smoothie (page 97)

Snack: 1 sliced orange and 2 hard-boiled eggs

Lunch: 12 grilled shrimp atop spinach salad with 2 tsp olive oil and 2 tsp lemon juice

Snack: ¼ cup/60 g pumpkin or sunflower seeds

Dinner: 5 Turkey Meatballs (page 83), steamed broccoli drizzled with 2 tsp olive oil and fresh lemon juice. Serve over *shirataki* or 100-percent buckwheat noodles, brown rice, or beans.

DAY 3

Breakfast: 2 slices Canadian bacon, 2 oz/55 g almond cheese with ½ cup/75 g blueberries

Snack: 1 apple sliced and smeared with 1 tbsp almond butter

Lunch: Crabmeat salad made with a 6-oz/170-g can of crabmeat, 1 chopped celery rib, 1 chopped scallion. Dress with 1 tbsp mayo and juice of ½ lemon. Serve inside ½ avocado. 1 cup/165 g strawberries. (Extra credit: Buy organic fresh or frozen strawberries.)

Snack: ¼ cup/30 g cashews, handful of grapes

Dinner: 6 oz/170 g buffalo burger (or substitute turkey for the buffalo) with roasted asparagus. (Wash 1 bunch of asparagus and place on a baking sheet. Drizzle with 2 tsp olive oil. Bake for 15 minutes at 350°F/180°C. Sprinkle fresh lemon juice and serve.) Serve with ½ cup/80 g sweet potato hash browns.

DAY 4

Breakfast: 6 oz/170 g canned wild Alaskan salmon mixed with 1 tsp mayo and 1 tsp apple cider vinegar. Serve with ½ avocado and ⅛ cantaloupe, sliced. (If you can't stomach salmon for breakfast, try 2 turkey sausages with sliced tomatoes and ½ cup/70 g berries or a Protein Smoothie; page 97.)

Snack: ¼ cup/30 g mixed raw nuts, ½ grapefruit

Lunch: 4 oz/115 g beef carpaccio topped with watercress and lemon, steamed artichokes, 1 cup/165 g strawberries for dessert

Snack: 2 oz/55 g sliced turkey breast rolled around ¼ avocado

Dinner: 6 oz/170 g grilled chicken, sliced yellow squash and zucchini sautéed with ½ cup/120 ml chicken broth and 1 clove crushed garlic. Finely grate almond cheese on top for a punch of flavor. Serve with ½ cup/100 g cooked wild rice.

DAY 5

Breakfast: Omelet: 2 whole eggs plus 2 whites, with ¼ cup/60 g each onions, spinach, and bell pepper. Serve with ⅛ cantaloupe, sliced.

Snack: 1 cup/165 g sliced strawberries topped with 2 tbsp slivered almonds

Lunch: Roast beef wrap (4 oz/115 g roast beef wrapped in lettuce) with ¼ avocado, side salad

Snack: 2 hard-boiled eggs and 5 Brazil nuts

Dinner: 6 oz/170 g Roasted Chicken (page 80), 1 cup/125 g steamed green beans. (Steam until al dente and bright green; remove beans and place in bowl of ice water for 3 minutes to stop cooking and retain green color. Then place back in steamer to keep warm.) Organic corn on the cob with 1 tsp butter.

DAY 6

Breakfast: 2 slices turkey bacon, 2 eggs, sunny-side up, cooked in 1 tsp butter, ½ cup/2 oz raspberries. (Extra credit: Use organic berries.)

Snack: 2 celery ribs smeared with 2 tbsp natural peanut butter

Lunch: 5 oz/140 g grilled chicken salad with 1 tbsp each fresh dill, chopped red onion, and olive oil over 2 cups/60 g raw spinach, 1 apple

Snack: Protein Smoothie (page 97)

Dinner: 6 oz/170 g filet mignon, 2 heads baby bok choy cooked in 1 tsp olive oil and sprinkled with sesame seeds, ½ cup/100 g wild rice cooked in chicken broth

DAY 7

Breakfast: 2 slices of turkey bacon, 2 oz/55 g almond cheese, 1 cup/ 150 g berries

Snack: Protein Smoothie (page 97) or 1 banana with 1 tbsp peanut butter. (Extra credit: Use natural peanut butter.)

Lunch: 6 oz/170 g buffalo burger (skip the bun) and a side salad with 1 tsp olive oil and 2 tsp vinegar; 1 pear for dessert

Snack: 2 oz/ 55 g sliced turkey breast rolled around ¼ avocado

Dinner: 6 oz/170 g red snapper with ½ cup/130 g sautéed white beans and 1 cup/155 g Brussels sprouts. (Wash and slice Brussels sprouts in half. Place in a medium bowl and toss with 2 tsp olive oil and a pinch of sea salt. Bake in a glass pan at 350°F/180°C for 45 minutes.)

DAY 8   **Breakfast:** 4 oz/110 g smoked salmon, ¼ avocado, 2-in/5-cm cantaloupe wedge

Snack: Protein Smoothie (page 97)

Lunch: Greek salad (hold the feta) with 5 oz/140 g grilled chicken, drizzled with oil and vinegar dressing; 1 peach for dessert

Snack: 2 oz/55 g sliced turkey breast rolled around ¼ avocado

Dinner: 5 oz/140 g lamb chop, sautéed broccoli rabe (1 bunch) sprinkled with sesame seeds, and ½ cup/60 g roasted baby potatoes. (Bake lamb chop for 15 to 20 minutes, depending on thickness, at 350°F/180°C on a baking sheet covered in foil or in a glass or enamel pan.)

DAY 9   **Breakfast:** 1 whole egg plus 3 egg whites scrambled with 1 oz/30 g shredded almond cheese and 1 tsp dried parsley. Serve with 1 cup/150 g fresh blueberries or cantaloupe.

Snack: 1 apple sliced and smeared with 1 tbsp almond butter

Lunch: 1 cup/245 g turkey chili, 1 cup/155 g steamed broccoli, 1 pear

Snack: 2 oz/55 g turkey jerky and 10 walnut halves

Dinner: 6 oz/170 g lamb or chicken, cubed and skewered with red onions, bell peppers, and cherry tomatoes. Brush with olive oil and bake for 25 minutes at 350°F/180°C. Serve atop arugula salad topped with 1 tsp pine nuts and ½ cup/95 g short-grain brown rice.

DAY 10   **Breakfast:** 4 oz/110 g smoked salmon, ¼ avocado, 1 sliced tomato, evenly distributed over 1 raw red bell pepper (halved) or Protein Smoothie (page 97)

Snack: 1 oz/30 g sweet potato chips and ¼ cup/60 g hummus

Lunch: 12 shrimp with 1 cup/190 g cooked rice or *shirataki* noodles tossed with 2 tbsp melted natural peanut butter and 2 tsp sesame oil with a side of sautéed bok choy

Snack: 2 oz/ 55 g sliced turkey breast rolled around ¼ avocado

Dinner: 6 oz/170 g chicken satay skewers, 3 vegetable dumplings, steamed vegetables

DAY 11   **Breakfast:** Protein Smoothie (page 97)

Snack: 2 oz/55 g turkey jerky and 1 orange

Lunch: 5 oz/140 g chicken brushed with pesto or salsa,
1 cup/155 g roasted carrots

Snack: 2 celery ribs with 2 tbsp natural peanut butter

Dinner: 6 oz/170 g wild Alaskan salmon (brush with 1 tsp pesto
sauce, bake at 350°F/180°C for 7 to 8 minutes) with 1 cup/180 g sautéed
spinach, 1 cup/120 g Sweet Potato "Fries" (page 92)

DAY 12   **Breakfast:** 3 scrambled eggs cooked in 1 tsp butter, side of "hash
browns" (leftover potatoes stir-fried with onions)

Snack: 1 apple sliced and smeared with 1 tbsp almond butter

Lunch: Turkey wrap (4 oz/115 g turkey wrapped in lettuce leaves) with
¼ avocado and ½ tomato, 1 cup/240 ml vegetable- or broth-based soup

Snack: Protein Smoothie (page 97)

Dinner: 6 oz/170 g turkey burger (no bun) with mustard and 1 tsp mayo.
Buy prewashed bags of spinach and make a side salad. Serve with
1 cup/120 g Sweet Potato "Fries" (page 92).

DAY 13   **Breakfast:** 4 oz/110 g smoked salmon with ¼ avocado and 1 tomato,
10 pecans

Snack: ¼ cup/30 g mixed raw nuts

Lunch: 5 oz/140 g turkey burger with 1 tbsp guacamole, red and yellow
tomato salad drizzled with 1 tsp olive oil and fresh basil, ½ cup/100 g
roasted butternut squash sprinkled with cinnamon

Snack: 2 oz/55 g slices beef jerky, sliced red bell pepper

Dinner: Omelet: 2 whole eggs plus 2 egg whites, ½ onion and ½ red
bell pepper. Serve with a side salad topped with ¼ cup/60 g chickpeas.

DAY 14   **Breakfast:** 2 chicken sausages with 1 sliced tomato and ½ cup/
80 g strawberries

Snack: Protein Smoothie (page 97)

Lunch: 12 grilled shrimp over ½ cup/95 g cooked brown rice with broccoli

Snack: 2 oz/55 g sliced turkey breast, 1 pear

Dinner: 6 oz/170 g buffalo burger with roasted asparagus and ½ cup/
100 g leftover butternut squash. (Wash 1 bunch of asparagus and place
on a baking sheet. Drizzle with 1 tsp olive oil. Bake for 15 minutes.
Sprinkle sesame seeds atop spears and serve.)

DAYS 15 TO 28: Repeat the cycle.

NUMBER

(3)

GORGEOUSLY BALANCED

If you are the kind of gal who stays centered by keeping things in balance, then this is the perfect plan for you. A mixture of proteins, carbs, and fats will keep your energy level up throughout the day and satisfy your need to have a little bit of everything on your plate. You may lose weight effortlessly on this plan, or you may simply maintain your weight. Either way, you will feel satiated after meals and not wanting more.

DAY 1

Breakfast: ½ cup/115 g cooked oats with 1 scoop vanilla whey powder, ½ cup/75 g berries

Snack: 2 celery ribs with 2 tbsp almond butter

Lunch: Turkey wrap (4 oz/115 g turkey wrapped in lettuce leaves) with ¼ avocado and ¼ tomato, 1 cup/240 ml vegetable or broth-based soup

Snack: ¼ cup/30 g mixed raw nuts and 1 orange

Dinner: 6 oz/170 g turkey burger with mustard and 1 tsp mayo, ½ sweet potato with 1 tsp butter. Buy prewashed bags of spinach and make a side salad.

DAY 2

Breakfast: Omelet: 2 scrambled eggs plus 2 egg whites, 1 chopped tomato, ¼ onion cooked in 1 tsp olive oil; ½ cup cooked oat bran; 1 cup/150 g fresh blueberries

Snack: ¼ cup/30 g mixed raw nuts

Lunch: Crabmeat salad made with a 6-oz/170-g can of crabmeat, 1 chopped celery rib, 1 chopped scallion. Dress with ¼ cup/55 g yogurt and juice of ½ lemon, and serve inside ½ avocado. Serve with 2 tbsp hummus and 1 cup/165 g strawberries. (Extra credit: Buy organic fresh or frozen strawberries.)

Snack: 2 oz/55 g sliced turkey breast rolled around ¼ avocado

Dinner: 6 oz/170 g grilled chicken, sliced yellow squash and zucchini sautéed with ½ cup/120 ml chicken broth and 1 clove crushed garlic, ½ cup/100 g cooked lentils

DAY 3   **Breakfast:** Protein Smoothie (page 97)

Snack: 10 almonds and 1 hard-boiled egg

Lunch: 12 grilled shrimp atop Caesar salad, ½ cup/100 g cooked lentils

Snack: 1 large raw carrot and 2 tbsp hummus

Dinner: 5 Turkey Meatballs (page 83), 1 baked potato with 1 tsp butter, ½ cup/90g sautéed spinach

DAY 4   **Breakfast:** 2 poached eggs and 2 oz/60 g smoked salmon with 1 sliced tomato and ¼ avocado

Snack: 1 apple sliced and smeared with 1 tbsp almond butter

Lunch: Large salad with 5 olives, 1 tomato, ½ orange bell pepper, ½ cucumber, 1 celery stalk. Add a 6-oz/170-g can of chicken (Extra credit: Have sardines, octopus, tuna, or salmon) and ½ cup/ 120 g canned, well-rinsed chickpeas. Drizzle with 2 tsp olive oil and fresh lemon juice.

Snack: ¼ cup/30 g raw pecans

Dinner: 6 oz/170 g buffalo burger (or substitute turkey for the buffalo) with ½ cup/100 g brown rice pilaf and roasted asparagus. (Wash 1 bunch of asparagus and place on a baking sheet. Drizzle with 2 tsp olive oil. Bake for 15 minutes at 350°F/180°C. Sprinkle fresh Parmesan atop spears and serve.)

DAY 5   **Breakfast:** 3 oz/85 g canned wild Alaskan salmon mixed with 1 tsp mayo and 1 tsp apple cider vinegar. Serve atop 2 Wasa crackers with 1-in/2.5-cm cantaloupe wedge. (If you can't stomach salmon for breakfast, try 2 turkey sausages with ½ cup/115 g cooked oats or a Protein Smoothie, page 97.)

Snack: ¼ cup/30 g mixed raw nuts

Lunch: Beef carpaccio salad topped with Parmesan and lemon, 1 slice pumpernickel bread, steamed artichokes

Snack: 2 oz/55 g sliced turkey breast rolled around ¼ avocado

Dinner: 6 oz/170 g grilled chicken, sliced yellow squash and zucchini sautéed with ½ cup/120 ml chicken broth and 1 clove crushed garlic, ½ cup/100 g cooked brown rice

DAY 6   **Breakfast:** ½ cup/115 g cooked rolled oats mixed with 1 heaping tsp whey protein, ½ sliced banana, 1 tbsp chopped walnuts, and ¼ cup almond milk

Snack: 1 cup/225 g plain yogurt with ½ cup/85 g sliced strawberries and 1 tbsp slivered almonds

Lunch: Roast beef wrap (4 oz/115 g roast beef wrapped in lettuce) with honey mustard, side salad

Snack: 1 hard-boiled egg and 1 banana

Dinner: 6 oz/170 g Roasted Chicken (page 80), ½ cup/4 oz cooked farro, 1 cup/125 g steamed green beans. (Steam until al dente and bright green; remove beans and place in bowl of ice water for 3 minutes to stop cooking and retain green color. Then place back in steamer to keep warm.)

DAY 7   **Breakfast:** 1 slice turkey bacon, 2 eggs, sunny-side up, cooked in 1 tsp butter, 1 cup/125 g raspberries. (Extra credit: Use organic berries.)

Snack: 2 celerys rib smeared with 2 tbsp natural peanut butter

Lunch: 5 oz/140 g grilled chicken salad with 1 tbsp each fresh dill, chopped red onion, garlic, and olive oil over 2 cups/60 g raw spinach sprinkled with ¼ cup/65 g canned and rinsed navy beans, 1 apple

Snack: 1 cup/225 g plain yogurt with ½ cup/85 g sliced strawberries and 1 tbsp slivered almonds

Dinner: 6 oz/170 g filet mignon, 2 heads baby bok choy cooked in 1 tsp olive oil and sprinkled with sesame seeds, ½ sweet potato with 1 tsp butter

DAY 8   **Breakfast:** 1 tbsp natural almond butter on 1 slice of high-fiber bread, 2 slices of turkey bacon

Snack: ½ serving Protein Smoothie (page 97) or 1 banana with 1 tbsp peanut butter. (Extra credit: Use natural peanut butter.)

Lunch: 5 oz/140 g buffalo burger (skip the bun) and a side salad with 1 tsp olive oil and 2 tsp vinegar

Snack: 2 oz/55 g sliced turkey breast rolled around ¼ avocado

Dinner: 6 oz/170 g red snapper with ½ cup/80 g cooked wild rice and 1 cup/155 g roasted Brussels sprouts. (Wash and slice Brussels sprouts in half. Place in a medium bowl and toss with 2 tsp olive oil and a pinch of sea salt. Bake in a glass pan at 350°F/180°C for 45 minutes.)

DAY 9

Breakfast: 3 oz/85 g smoked salmon, ¼ cup slow-cooking oatmeal with ¼ cup/35 g blueberries or ½ cup cooked rolled oats mixed with 1 tsp whey protein, ½ sliced banana, 1 tbsp chopped walnuts, and ¼ cup/60 g almond milk

Snack: ½ cup/115 g cottage cheese with ¼ cup/35 g blueberries

Lunch: Greek salad with 3 oz/85 g grilled chicken and 2 tbsp hummus, drizzled with 2 tsp Italian dressing

Snack: 2 slices turkey breast rolled around ¼ avocado

Dinner: 5 oz/140 g lamb chop, ½ small sweet potato with 1 tsp butter, 2 heads sautéed baby bok choy sprinkled with sesame seeds. (Bake lamb chop for 15 to 20 minutes, depending on thickness, at 350°F/180°C on a baking sheet covered in foil or in a glass or enamel pan.)

DAY 10

Breakfast: 2 slices Canadian bacon, ½ cup/115 g cottage cheese sprinkled with ½ cup/75 g blueberries

Snack: 1 apple sliced and smeared with 1 tbsp almond butter

Lunch: 1 cup/245 g turkey chili served with a dollop of plain yogurt, 1 cup/155 g steamed broccoli, 1 pear

Snack: 1 cup/225 g plain yogurt with ½ cup/80 g sliced strawberries and 1 tbsp slivered almonds

Dinner: 6 oz/170 g lamb or chicken, cubed and skewered with red onions, bell peppers, and cherry tomatoes. Brush with olive oil and bake for 25 minutes at 350°F/180°C. Serve atop ¼ cup/40 g of tabouli salad, 1 cup/20 g arugula, 1 tsp pine nuts.

DAY 11   **Breakfast:** 4 oz/110 g smoked salmon, ¼ avocado, 1 sliced tomato, evenly distributed over 2 rye Wasa crackers or Protein Smoothie (page 97)

Snack: ½ cup/115 g cottage cheese with ¼ cup/35 g blueberries

Lunch: 1 cup/245 g ginger-carrot soup (broth based), 4 oz/115 g beef carpaccio salad with lemon and Parmesan, ½ cup/100 g cooked lentils

Snack: 1 sliced orange and 1 hard-boiled egg

Dinner: 6 oz/170 g chicken satay skewers, 3 vegetable dumplings, steamed vegetables

DAY 12   **Breakfast:** Protein Smoothie (page 97)

Snack: 1 cup/225 g plain yogurt with ½ cup/85 g sliced strawberries and 1 tbsp slivered almonds

Lunch: 4 oz/115 g chicken brushed with pesto or salsa, 1 cup/205 g roasted butternut squash, 1 cup/155 g roasted carrots

Snack: 1 apple sliced and smeared with 1 tbsp almond butter

Dinner: 6 oz/170 g wild Alaskan salmon (brush with 1 tsp pesto sauce, bake at 350°F/180°C for 7 to 8 minutes) with ½ cup/100 g cooked lentils (you can use canned lentils to save time) and 1 cup/180 g sautéed spinach

DAY 13   **Breakfast:** 1 cup/225 g plain yogurt, ½ cup/85 g strawberries, 1 tbsp ground flaxseeds, 1 tbsp chopped pecans (Extra credit: Use organic yogurt.)

Snack: ¼ cup/30 g mixed raw nuts

Lunch: 5 oz/140 g turkey burger with 1 tbsp guacamole, red and yellow tomato salad drizzled with 1 tsp olive oil and fresh basil, 1 small ear corn on the cob

Snack: 1 sliced red bell pepper with ¼ cup/60 g hummus

Dinner: Omelet: Scramble 2 whole eggs plus 2 egg whites, ½ onion, and ½ red bell pepper. Serve with a side salad and a slice of buttered hemp bread.

DAY 14

Breakfast: ½ cup/115 g cooked oats served with ¼ cup/40 g sliced strawberries, 1 tbsp crushed pecans, 1 tbsp ground flaxseeds, and ½ cup/120 ml 2-percent milk.

Snack: 1 hard-boiled egg and 1 banana

Lunch: Beet and goat cheese salad with walnuts and 12 grilled shrimp

Snack: 2 oz/55 g sliced turkey breast, 5 almonds, 1 pear

Dinner: 6 oz/170 g buffalo burger with ½ cup/95 g brown rice pilaf and roasted asparagus. (Wash 1 bunch asparagus and place on a baking sheet. Drizzle with 2 tsp olive oil. Bake for 15 minutes at 350°F/180°C. Sprinkle fresh Parmesan atop spears and serve.)

DAYS 15 TO 28: Repeat the cycle.

LEAN–BODY DIET

The goal of this diet is to bust up stubborn body fat by controlling insulin output (and ideally minimizing it) throughout the day. This meal plan is rich in protein and fiber to help you burn body fat while preserving lean muscle. Carbs are doled out at dinner to counterbalance cortisol and help you sleep. Give your body at least 5 to 7 days to adjust to this plan. Warning: Once you see the transformative effects of a lean-body diet coupled with weight-based workouts, you may never go back to your old habits! Make sure that one night per week you indulge in your favorite meal and have a glass of wine or dessert. Then get right back on the wagon. Have fun!

DAY 1

Breakfast: 4 to 6 egg whites (this equals 1 to 1½ cup packaged egg whites) with 1 sliced tomato and a handful of raw pecans

Snack: Protein Smoothie (page 97)

Lunch: 2 grilled chicken breasts over a large salad with balsamic vinegar

Snack: 3-oz/85-g can of low-mercury tuna or salmon, 2 celery ribs

Dinner: 5 oz/140 g filet mignon, spinach salad with lemon juice and a sprinkle of Parmesan, 8 asparagus spears, baked sweet potato with 1 tsp butter

DAY 2

Breakfast: 2 turkey sausages, 1 sliced raw bell pepper, ¼ cup/60 g raw cashews

Snack: 2 oz/55 g sliced turkey breast with mustard, 1 small apple

Lunch: 6-oz/170-g can of salmon mixed with 1 tsp olive oil and 1 tbsp apple cider vinegar, served with asparagus and grilled vegetables

Snack: 1 apple and 10 almonds

Dinner: 6 oz/170 g buffalo burger, steamed spinach with lemon juice, ¼ cup/50 g cooked lentils

DAY 3

Breakfast: ½ grapefruit, 4-egg-white omelet with tomatoes, mushrooms, onions, and 1 oz/30 g grated almond cheese

Snack: Protein Smoothie (page 97)

Lunch: Large spinach salad with tomatoes, shredded cabbage, 6 oz/170 g cubed chicken and ham, drizzled with 1 tsp olive oil and 1 tbsp balsamic vinegar

Snack: 2 oz/55 g sliced turkey breast with mustard, handful of cherry tomatoes

Dinner: 5 Turkey Meatballs (page 83) served with ¼ cup/50 g brown rice and grilled zucchini

DAY 4

Breakfast: 4 to 6 oz/110 to 170 g smoked salmon with ⅛ avocado, 1 tomato, and 1 cup/150 g berries

Snack: 1 handful of pecans

Lunch: 6 oz/170 g low-mercury tuna fish with 1 tsp olive oil and 1 tbsp apple cider vinegar, steamed broccoli and asparagus

Snack: 8 oz/235 ml green vegetable juice and a protein bar

Dinner: 10 broiled scallops with rosemary, steamed artichokes, ½ cup/100 g lentils with sautéed onions

DAY 5

Breakfast: 6 oz/170 g leftover chicken, turkey, or other lean meat smeared with mustard or tomato sauce, ½ grapefruit

Snack: 2 celery ribs smeared with 2 tbsp natural peanut butter

Lunch: 6 oz/170 g turkey burger wrapped in lettuce with tomatoes, a dollop of guacamole, sliced peppers (raw or roasted), and baby carrots

Snack: Protein Smoothie (page 97)

Dinner: 6 oz/170 g filet mignon with ½ baked sweet potato with 1 tsp butter, shredded zucchini sautéed with ½ cup/120 ml chicken broth and topped with shaved Parmesan

DAY 6

Breakfast: Omelet: 2 whole eggs plus 2 to 4 egg whites, mushrooms, onions, peppers, and 1 oz/30 g almond cheese

Snack: Protein Smoothie (page 97)

Lunch: Large bowl of tomato soup (no added sugar), 6-oz/170-g can of salmon with 1 tsp olive oil and 1 tbsp apple cider vinegar atop large spinach salad with mushrooms, red onions, cherry tomatoes, cucumbers, and celery

Snack: 8 oz/235 ml green vegetable juice and a protein bar

Dinner: "Slop": Caramelize 1 yellow onion in 2 tsp butter. Add in 1 lb/ 455 g ground buffalo meat and brown. Add in 1 jar tomato sauce, a 15-oz/430-g can of chickpeas or other beans, and 1 tsp each cumin, onion powder, and garlic powder. Simmer for 30 minutes on low heat. Before serving, add 1 bag of prewashed spinach and stir until lightly wilted. Serve slop in large bowls with 1 oz/30 g grated almond cheese on top.

DAY 7

Breakfast: 2 turkey sausages, 1 sliced bell pepper, ¼ cup/60 g raw cashews

Snack: ½ grapefruit, 1 oz/30 g walnuts (about 15 halves)

Lunch: Manhattan clam chowder, 6 oz/170 g smoked salmon topped with arugula and shaved Parmesan, drizzled with 1 tsp olive oil and fresh lemon juice

Snack: Protein Smoothie (page 97)

Dinner: 6 oz/170 g turkey burger. Serve with sautéed spinach (1 bag prewashed spinach sautéed in chicken broth and sprinkled with onion powder). Optional: 1 cup/120 g Sweet Potato "Fries" (page 92).

DAY 8

Breakfast: 6 oz/170 g steak, ¼ avocado, 1 sliced tomato

Snack: 2 oz/55 g almond cheese and 1 apple

Lunch: 5 oz/140 g buffalo burger chopped up in a spinach salad with tomatoes, carrots, shredded cabbage, 1 tsp olive oil, and 1 tbsp balsamic vinegar

Snack: 2 oz/55 g turkey slices with mustard, 1 handful baby carrots

Dinner: Chicken fajitas: 6 oz/170 g chicken, ½ green bell pepper and ¼ onion sautéed in 1 tsp olive oil and chicken broth, salsa; 1 oz/30 g almond cheese and dollop of guacamole; served atop a low-carb, high-fiber tortilla.

DAY 9

Breakfast: 1 slice turkey bacon, 3 whole eggs plus 3 egg whites scrambled with tomatoes and broccoli

Snack: 1 apple smeared with 1 tbsp peanut butter

Lunch: Chicken salad: 6-oz/170-g can of chicken mixed with 1 tsp olive oil, 1 tbsp balsamic vinegar. Serve atop chopped romaine lettuce, shredded carrots, shredded cabbage, and grape tomatoes.

Snack: 1 chicken breast with mustard, cherry tomatoes and baby carrots

Dinner: 6 oz/170 g broiled wild Alaskan salmon, mashed cauliflower, chickpeas sautéed in chicken broth with onion powder, garlic powder, and dried parsley. (To make mashed cauliflower, steam 1 head of cauliflower in 2 cups/480 ml chicken broth until fork-tender [about 20 minutes]. Place cauliflower and remaining liquid in a blender with ¼ cup olive oil. Pulse until desired consistency is reached. Leftovers will keep in fridge for up to 5 days.)

DAY 10

Breakfast: 6 oz/170 g chicken breast with salsa, 10 Brazil nuts

Snack: ½ grapefruit and 1 oz/30 g pecans (about 15 halves)

Lunch: Turkey wrap (6 oz/165 g turkey wrapped in lettuce leaves). Serve with cabbage slaw.

Snack: 3-oz/85-g can of low-mercury tuna, carrot and celery sticks

Dinner: 12 shrimp sautéed with ½ cup/90 g white beans in a mixture of 2 tbsp fresh lemon juice, ½ cup/120 ml chicken broth, 1 clove crushed garlic, and 1 tsp olive oil. After the shrimp is cooked, remove from pan and cover. Continue to heat chicken broth mixture over low heat for another 7 minutes, until it reduces slightly. Sauté spinach with 1 tsp olive oil. Serve shrimp, with sauce on top, atop wilted spinach.

DAY 11

Breakfast: Egg-white frittata: Cook 4 to 6 egg whites in a skillet in 1 tsp olive oil until the whites begin to firm up. Add ½ cup/15 g packed raw spinach, ¼ cup/10 g sliced mushrooms, ½ diced red bell pepper. Continue cooking until the whites are completely firm. Serve with ½ baked sweet potato cut into cubes and ½ cup/75 g berries.

Snack: 1 pear and 2 ham slices

Lunch: 12 grilled shrimp atop arugula with cherry tomatoes, steamed asparagus (8 spears). Grate fresh Parmesan on top and drizzle 1 tsp olive oil and 1 tbsp balsamic vinegar.

Snack: Unlimited raw vegetables and 4 oz/115 g turkey breast

Dinner: 6 oz/170 g Roasted Chicken (page 80). Halve 1 cup/90 g Brussels sprouts and peel outer leaves off core; place in 1-qt/960-ml saucepan. Steam for 3 minutes on high and remove from heat. Toss with 1 tsp olive oil and a dash of onion powder and sea salt. Chop 5 pecans and sprinkle on top. Serve with ½ cup/100 g brown rice.

DAY 12   Breakfast: 3 oz/85 g smoked salmon scrambled with 3 egg whites, 5 almonds

Snack: 1 scoop whey protein powder, ½ banana, 1 cup almond milk, dash of cinnamon, blended with ice

Lunch: 2 grilled chicken breasts, large salad with lettuce, celery, carrots, cabbage, and tomatoes. Drizzle with 1 tsp olive oil and 1 tbsp balsamic vinegar.

Snack: 3-oz/85-g can of salmon with 1 tsp olive oil, baby carrots

Dinner: 5 Turkey Meatballs (page 83). Serve with ½ cup/100 g brown rice and grated zucchini sautéed in ½ cup/120 ml chicken broth and topped with grated Parmesan.

DAY 13   Breakfast: 2 whole eggs plus 2 to 4 egg whites scrambled with spinach, mushrooms, and onions; ½ grapefruit

Snack: 1 scoop whey protein, 1 tbsp ground flaxseeds, 1 cup/240 g almond milk, ½ cup/75 g frozen berries, dash of cinnamon, blended with ice

Lunch: 3 leftover Turkey Meatballs, 1 cup/155 g steamed broccoli, ½ cup/100 g cooked lentils

Snack: Leftover chicken drumstick with celery and carrots

Dinner: 10 broiled scallops with rosemary, roasted zucchini, spinach salad with 1 tsp olive oil and 1 tbsp fresh lemon juice, ½ cup/100 g cooked lentils

DAY 14   **Breakfast:** 3 oz/85 g smoked salmon, 2 hard-boiled eggs, tomato and cucumber salad

Snack: 1 handful walnuts, small apple

Lunch: 5 oz/140 g broiled salmon, shredded sautéed bok choy, sprinkled with sesame seeds

Snack: 1 bell pepper stuffed with 3 oz/85 g canned low-mercury tuna fish

Dinner: 6 oz/170 g broiled filet mignon with spinach sautéed in chicken broth, 8 asparagus spears, ½ cup/95 g cooked quinoa

DAYS 15 TO 28: Repeat cycle.

SHOPPING LIST

To get you started, here is a basic list of items you should have on hand. Whenever possible, buy organic. When you get home from the grocery store, freeze your meats so you can just pull them out of the freezer to defrost the day you're ready to eat them. Double-check the meal plan you're intending to follow (see pages 100–125) to make sure to stock up on all the foods listed in your plan. Remember, setting yourself up for success means no excuses!

PROTEINS

You need 4–6 oz/115–170 g of protein per meal to sustain muscle mass, burn body fat, boost energy, balance blood sugar and hormones, and promote bone density.

- ◯ Grass-fed beef
- ◯ Grass-fed lamb
- ◯ Chicken
- ◯ Turkey
- ◯ Cornish hen, pheasant, or any other wild game
- ◯ Buffalo
- ◯ Venison
- ◯ Ostrich
- ◯ Fish
- ◯ Eggs
- ◯ Greek yogurt
- ◯ Almond cheese
- ◯ Whey, pea, or rice protein powder
- ◯ Protein bars

CARBOHYDRATES

We all need some amount of carbohydrates each day, but the amount needed varies per person. For one month, try using only fruits and vegetables as your carbo-hydrates. Then slowly add back ½ cup/40 g cooked complex carbohydrates each day to determine the amount that is right for you.

- ◯ Fresh fruits (apples, small bananas, grapefruits, oranges, blackberries, blueberries, cantaloupe, raspberries, strawberries)
- ◯ Fresh vegetables (any and all!; artichokes, broccoli, Brussels sprouts, cabbage, cauliflower, carrots, cucumbers, eggplant, green beans, kale, peppers, spinach, tomatoes, zucchini)
- ◯ Rolled oats and oat bran
- ◯ Sweet potatoes
- ◯ Winter squash (acorn, butternut, spaghetti)
- ◯ Barley
- ◯ Brown rice
- ◯ Beans (dry or canned)
- ◯ Lentils (dry or canned)
- ◯ Quinoa
- ◯ Amaranth
- ◯ Millet
- ◯ Buckwheat (kasha)
- ◯ Hemp bread
- ◯ Hummus

FATS

Fats are a crucial part of sustaining health and well-being. Fats are powerful regulators of inflammation and will control how our bodies burn or store fat. The right fats will heal you and help eliminate heart disease, diabetes, osteoporosis, joint pain, and obesity. The wrong fats will give you all the diseases listed above and then some.

- ○ Butter
- ○ Avocado
- ○ Raw nuts and seeds
- ○ Raw nut butters
- ○ Tahini
- ○ Olives

- ○ Olive oil
- ○ Grapeseed oil
- ○ Coconut oil
- ○ Coconut flakes (unsweetened)
- ○ Flax oil (store in the refrigerator)
- ○ Ground flaxseeds
  (store in the freezer)

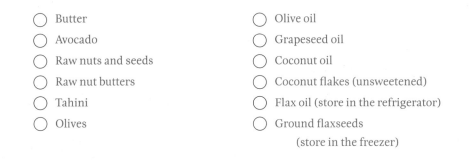

Fast Food 101

Keep these items in your fridge and you're ready to rock out your lunch: organic celery, organic mixed greens (prewashed), shredded cabbage, grape tomatoes, and rinsed canned chicken. Place the items on a large plate, drizzle with 1 tsp olive oil and 1 tbsp raw cider vinegar, and toss. Lunch is served!

FOOD DIARY

Turn the page to get a glimpse of your food log pages, and embark on your transformative body journey. These pages are designed to help you easily keep track of what you're eating and get a leg up on leanness. Self-enlightenment is the greatest perk of owning your actions, and these log pages will give you the tools to reach your goals. Putting pen to paper will awaken your senses and bring your eating to a conscious level. So grab a pen, check into your mind, and get writing. This time is insanely ripe with potential. Shine on!

Keeping track of what you eat is fairly straightforward; the thing that sometimes trips people up is that they try to write down their meals after they've eaten or at the end of the day. Many clients tell me they're too busy during the day to keep a food log, so they try to write it all down at night before bed. In my experience, this leaves too much margin for error. In order to keep your eating clean and tight you need to record the deed as it's done. For people who find it challenging to stay on track, I recommend writing what you eat *before* you eat it. That way you get it over and done with, and you'll keep your focus razor sharp. The only way to hit the target is by aiming straight ahead! Keep this diary in a prominent place in the kitchen, where you eat most often, or, better yet, carry it with you in your bag.

When logging your food, write down what you eat and how much of it you're eating. If you're at home, put your measuring cups to good use when counting your servings of starch—measure out cooked starches before you put them on your plate. If you're out on the town, use large tablespoons to measure out your starch; 2 tbsp equals $\frac{1}{8}$ cup of a grain or starch. For proteins, a portion the size of the palm of your hand is usually an appropriate single serving. And with salad dressings and added fats, ask for them on the side and then serve yourself 1 tsp with plenty of lemon juice or vinegar. I recommend taking some time to practice eyeballing what a normal portion size is; this is a skill that takes a bit of time to master. Also, remember to listen to your hunger/fullness cues; you may fill up long before your meal is done, in which case you can bring your leftovers home! Conversely, if you've had a hard workout and are extra hungry you may need to ramp up the protein and vegetables to give your body all that it needs.

Check in with yourself before and during meals to determine your hunger levels. Rate your hunger on a scale of 1 to 10, where a 1 is ravenous and a 10 is overstuffed. Ideally, you will start eating at a 2 or 3 and stop somewhere near 5, when you are satisfied. Don't let yourself get too hungry or too full; somewhere in between is just right. As you experiment, you will find that you are a work in progress, but you will hit your stride with practiced mindfulness!

Today's Date: *January 1*

EXERCISE

10 min warmup sprints on treadmill
30 mins weights

BREAKFAST

2 hard-boiled eggs, 1/2 cup cooked
oats, 1/2 cup cherries, coffee w/cream

SNACK

apple + peanut butter

LUNCH

salad bar: chicken, spinach, avocado,
chickpeas, tomatoes w/balsamic vinegar

SNACK

office party:
small piece of cake and skinny latte

DINNER

sushi -
one California roll, salmon tartare,
miso soup, side salad + 1 glass cold sake

SPLURGE

DAILY NEEDS

WATER	
✓ 8 oz/240 ml	✓ 8 oz/240 ml
✓ 8 oz/240 ml	✓ 8 oz/240 ml
✓ 8 oz/240 ml	✓ 8 oz/240 ml
✓ 8 oz/240 ml	○ 8 oz/240 ml
○ 8 oz/240 ml	○ 8 oz/240 ml

PROTEIN	
✓ 4 oz/115 g	✓ 4 oz/115 g
✓ 4 oz/115 g	○ 4 oz/115 g

FAT	
✓ 1 tbsp	✓ 1 tbsp
✓ 1 tbsp	

LOW-SUGAR VEGGIES	
✓ 1/2 cup/50 g	✓ 1/2 cup/50 g
✓ 1/2 cup/50 g	✓ 1/2 cup/50 g
○ 1/2 cup/50 g	○ 1/2 cup/50 g

COMPLEX CARBS	
✓ 1/2 cup/50 g	✓ 1/2 cup/50 g

LOW-SUGAR FRUITS	
✓ 1/2 cup/50 g	✓ 1/2 cup/50 g
○ 1/2 cup/50 g	○ 1/2 cup/50 g

CHECK IN

Did you feel satisfied after each meal?

Still hungry after workout-had apple 1 hour later.

Did you have cravings today?

No

What's one thing you were grateful for today?

Quality time with friends.

Today's Date:

EXERCISE

LUNCH

BREAKFAST

SNACK

SNACK

DINNER

DAILY NEEDS

WATER
- ◯ 8 oz/240 ml
- ◯ 8 oz/240 ml
- ◯ 8 oz/240 ml
- ◯ 8 oz/240 ml
- ◯ 8 oz/240 ml

- ◯ 8 oz/240 ml
- ◯ 8 oz/240 ml
- ◯ 8 oz/240 ml
- ◯ 8 oz/240 ml
- ◯ 8 oz/240 ml

PROTEIN
- ◯ 4 oz/115 g
- ◯ 4 oz/115 g

- ◯ 4 oz/115 g
- ◯ 4 oz/115 g

FAT
- ◯ 1 tbsp
- ◯ 1 tbsp

- ◯ 1 tbsp

LOW-SUGAR VEGGIES
- ◯ ½ cup/50 g
- ◯ ½ cup/50 g
- ◯ ½ cup/50 g

- ◯ ½ cup/50 g
- ◯ ½ cup/50 g
- ◯ ½ cup/50 g

COMPLEX CARBS
- ◯ ½ cup/50 g

- ◯ ½ cup/50 g

LOW-SUGAR FRUITS
- ◯ ½ cup/50 g
- ◯ ½ cup/50 g

- ◯ ½ cup/50 g
- ◯ ½ cup/50 g

CHECK IN

Did you feel satisfied after each meal?

Did you have cravings today?

What's one thing you were grateful for today?

Today's Date:

EXERCISE

LUNCH

BREAKFAST

SNACK

SNACK

DINNER

DAILY NEEDS

WATER

○ 8 oz/240 ml ○ 8 oz/240 ml
○ 8 oz/240 ml ○ 8 oz/240 ml
○ 8 oz/240 ml ○ 8 oz/240 ml
○ 8 oz/240 ml ○ 8 oz/240 ml
○ 8 oz/240 ml ○ 8 oz/240 ml

PROTEIN

○ 4 oz/115 g ○ 4 oz/115 g
○ 4 oz/115 g ○ 4 oz/115 g

FAT

○ 1 tbsp ○ 1 tbsp
○ 1 tbsp

LOW-SUGAR VEGGIES

○ ½ cup/50 g ○ ½ cup/50 g
○ ½ cup/50 g ○ ½ cup/50 g
○ ½ cup/50 g ○ ½ cup/50 g

COMPLEX CARBS

○ ½ cup/50 g ○ ½ cup/50 g

LOW-SUGAR FRUITS

○ ½ cup/50 g ○ ½ cup/50 g
○ ½ cup/50 g ○ ½ cup/50 g

CHECK IN

Did you feel satisfied after each meal?

Did you have cravings today?

What's one thing you were grateful for today?

Today's Date:

FOOD AND FITNESS LOG

EXERCISE

LUNCH

BREAKFAST

SNACK

SNACK

DINNER

DAILY NEEDS

WATER
- ◯ 8 oz/240 ml
- ◯ 8 oz/240 ml
- ◯ 8 oz/240 ml
- ◯ 8 oz/240 ml
- ◯ 8 oz/240 ml

- ◯ 8 oz/240 ml
- ◯ 8 oz/240 ml
- ◯ 8 oz/240 ml
- ◯ 8 oz/240 ml
- ◯ 8 oz/240 ml

PROTEIN
- ◯ 4 oz/115 g
- ◯ 4 oz/115 g

- ◯ 4 oz/115 g
- ◯ 4 oz/115 g

FAT
- ◯ 1 tbsp
- ◯ 1 tbsp

- ◯ 1 tbsp

LOW-SUGAR VEGGIES
- ◯ ½ cup/50 g
- ◯ ½ cup/50 g
- ◯ ½ cup/50 g

- ◯ ½ cup/50 g
- ◯ ½ cup/50 g
- ◯ ½ cup/50 g

COMPLEX CARBS
- ◯ ½ cup/50 g
- ◯ ½ cup/50 g

LOW-SUGAR FRUITS
- ◯ ½ cup/50 g
- ◯ ½ cup/50 g

- ◯ ½ cup/50 g
- ◯ ½ cup/50 g

CHECK IN

Did you feel satisfied after each meal?

Did you have cravings today?

What's one thing you were grateful for today?

Today's Date:

EXERCISE

LUNCH

BREAKFAST

SNACK

SNACK

DINNER

DAILY NEEDS

WATER

- ◯ 8 oz/240 ml
- ◯ 8 oz/240 ml
- ◯ 8 oz/240 ml
- ◯ 8 oz/240 ml
- ◯ 8 oz/240 ml

- ◯ 8 oz/240 ml
- ◯ 8 oz/240 ml
- ◯ 8 oz/240 ml
- ◯ 8 oz/240 ml
- ◯ 8 oz/240 ml

PROTEIN

- ◯ 4 oz/115 g
- ◯ 4 oz/115 g

- ◯ 4 oz/115 g
- ◯ 4 oz/115 g

FAT

- ◯ 1 tbsp
- ◯ 1 tbsp

- ◯ 1 tbsp

LOW-SUGAR VEGGIES

- ◯ ½ cup/50 g
- ◯ ½ cup/50 g
- ◯ ½ cup/50 g

- ◯ ½ cup/50 g
- ◯ ½ cup/50 g
- ◯ ½ cup/50 g

COMPLEX CARBS

- ◯ ½ cup/50 g

- ◯ ½ cup/50 g

LOW-SUGAR FRUITS

- ◯ ½ cup/50 g
- ◯ ½ cup/50 g

- ◯ ½ cup/50 g
- ◯ ½ cup/50 g

CHECK IN

Did you feel satisfied after each meal?

Did you have cravings today?

What's one thing you were grateful for today?

Today's Date:

FOOD AND FITNESS LOG

EXERCISE

LUNCH

BREAKFAST

SNACK

SNACK

DINNER

SPLURGE

DAILY NEEDS

WATER
- ○ 8 oz/240 ml
- ○ 8 oz/240 ml
- ○ 8 oz/240 ml
- ○ 8 oz/240 ml
- ○ 8 oz/240 ml
- ○ 8 oz/240 ml
- ○ 8 oz/240 ml
- ○ 8 oz/240 ml
- ○ 8 oz/240 ml
- ○ 8 oz/240 ml

PROTEIN
- ○ 4 oz/115 g
- ○ 4 oz/115 g
- ○ 4 oz/115 g
- ○ 4 oz/115 g

FAT
- ○ 1 tbsp
- ○ 1 tbsp
- ○ 1 tbsp

LOW-SUGAR VEGGIES
- ○ ½ cup/50 g
- ○ ½ cup/50 g
- ○ ½ cup/50 g
- ○ ½ cup/50 g
- ○ ½ cup/50 g
- ○ ½ cup/50 g

COMPLEX CARBS
- ○ ½ cup/50 g
- ○ ½ cup/50 g

LOW-SUGAR FRUITS
- ○ ½ cup/50 g
- ○ ½ cup/50 g
- ○ ½ cup/50 g
- ○ ½ cup/50 g

CHECK IN

Did you feel satisfied after each meal?

Did you have cravings today?

What's one thing you were grateful for today?

Today's Date:

EXERCISE

LUNCH

BREAKFAST

SNACK

SNACK

DINNER

DAILY NEEDS

WATER

○ 8 oz/240 ml   ○ 8 oz/240 ml

○ 8 oz/240 ml   ○ 8 oz/240 ml

○ 8 oz/240 ml   ○ 8 oz/240 ml

○ 8 oz/240 ml   ○ 8 oz/240 ml

○ 8 oz/240 ml   ○ 8 oz/240 ml

PROTEIN

○ 4 oz/115 g   ○ 4 oz/115 g

○ 4 oz/115 g   ○ 4 oz/115 g

FAT

○ 1 tbsp   ○ 1 tbsp

○ 1 tbsp

LOW-SUGAR VEGGIES

○ ½ cup/50 g   ○ ½ cup/50 g

○ ½ cup/50 g   ○ ½ cup/50 g

○ ½ cup/50 g   ○ ½ cup/50 g

COMPLEX CARBS

○ ½ cup/50 g   ○ ½ cup/50 g

LOW-SUGAR FRUITS

○ ½ cup/50 g   ○ ½ cup/50 g

○ ½ cup/50 g   ○ ½ cup/50 g

CHECK IN

Did you feel satisfied after each meal?

Did you have cravings today?

What's one thing you were grateful for today?

Today's Date:

FOOD AND FITNESS LOG

EXERCISE

LUNCH

BREAKFAST

SNACK

SNACK

DINNER

DAILY NEEDS

WATER
- ◯ 8 oz/240 ml
- ◯ 8 oz/240 ml
- ◯ 8 oz/240 ml
- ◯ 8 oz/240 ml
- ◯ 8 oz/240 ml
- ◯ 8 oz/240 ml
- ◯ 8 oz/240 ml
- ◯ 8 oz/240 ml
- ◯ 8 oz/240 ml
- ◯ 8 oz/240 ml

PROTEIN
- ◯ 4 oz/115 g
- ◯ 4 oz/115 g
- ◯ 4 oz/115 g
- ◯ 4 oz/115 g

FAT
- ◯ 1 tbsp
- ◯ 1 tbsp
- ◯ 1 tbsp

LOW-SUGAR VEGGIES
- ◯ ½ cup/50 g
- ◯ ½ cup/50 g
- ◯ ½ cup/50 g
- ◯ ½ cup/50 g
- ◯ ½ cup/50 g
- ◯ ½ cup/50 g

COMPLEX CARBS
- ◯ ½ cup/50 g
- ◯ ½ cup/50 g

LOW-SUGAR FRUITS
- ◯ ½ cup/50 g
- ◯ ½ cup/50 g
- ◯ ½ cup/50 g
- ◯ ½ cup/50 g

CHECK IN

Did you feel satisfied after each meal?

Did you have cravings today?

What's one thing you were grateful for today?

Today's Date:

EXERCISE

LUNCH

BREAKFAST

SNACK

SNACK

DINNER

DAILY NEEDS

WATER
- ◯ 8 oz/240 ml ◯ 8 oz/240 ml
- ◯ 8 oz/240 ml ◯ 8 oz/240 ml
- ◯ 8 oz/240 ml ◯ 8 oz/240 ml
- ◯ 8 oz/240 ml ◯ 8 oz/240 ml
- ◯ 8 oz/240 ml ◯ 8 oz/240 ml

PROTEIN
- ◯ 4 oz/115 g ◯ 4 oz/115 g
- ◯ 4 oz/115 g ◯ 4 oz/115 g

FAT
- ◯ 1 tbsp ◯ 1 tbsp
- ◯ 1 tbsp

LOW-SUGAR VEGGIES
- ◯ ½ cup/50 g ◯ ½ cup/50 g
- ◯ ½ cup/50 g ◯ ½ cup/50 g
- ◯ ½ cup/50 g ◯ ½ cup/50 g

COMPLEX CARBS
- ◯ ½ cup/50 g ◯ ½ cup/50 g

LOW-SUGAR FRUITS
- ◯ ½ cup/50 g ◯ ½ cup/50 g
- ◯ ½ cup/50 g ◯ ½ cup/50 g

CHECK IN

Did you feel satisfied after each meal?

Did you have cravings today?

What's one thing you were grateful for today?

Today's Date:

FOOD AND FITNESS LOG

EXERCISE

LUNCH

BREAKFAST

SNACK

SNACK

DINNER

DAILY NEEDS

WATER
- ◯ 8 oz/240 ml
- ◯ 8 oz/240 ml
- ◯ 8 oz/240 ml
- ◯ 8 oz/240 ml
- ◯ 8 oz/240 ml
- ◯ 8 oz/240 ml
- ◯ 8 oz/240 ml
- ◯ 8 oz/240 ml
- ◯ 8 oz/240 ml
- ◯ 8 oz/240 ml

PROTEIN
- ◯ 4 oz/115 g
- ◯ 4 oz/115 g
- ◯ 4 oz/115 g
- ◯ 4 oz/115 g

FAT
- ◯ 1 tbsp
- ◯ 1 tbsp
- ◯ 1 tbsp

LOW-SUGAR VEGGIES
- ◯ ½ cup/50 g
- ◯ ½ cup/50 g
- ◯ ½ cup/50 g
- ◯ ½ cup/50 g
- ◯ ½ cup/50 g
- ◯ ½ cup/50 g

COMPLEX CARBS
- ◯ ½ cup/50 g
- ◯ ½ cup/50 g

LOW-SUGAR FRUITS
- ◯ ½ cup/50 g
- ◯ ½ cup/50 g
- ◯ ½ cup/50 g
- ◯ ½ cup/50 g

CHECK IN

Did you feel satisfied after each meal?

Did you have cravings today?

What's one thing you were grateful for today?

Today's Date:

EXERCISE

LUNCH

BREAKFAST

SNACK

SNACK

DINNER

DAILY NEEDS

WATER		
	◯ 8 oz/240 ml	◯ 8 oz/240 ml
	◯ 8 oz/240 ml	◯ 8 oz/240 ml
	◯ 8 oz/240 ml	◯ 8 oz/240 ml
	◯ 8 oz/240 ml	◯ 8 oz/240 ml
	◯ 8 oz/240 ml	◯ 8 oz/240 ml

PROTEIN		
	◯ 4 oz/115 g	◯ 4 oz/115 g
	◯ 4 oz/115 g	◯ 4 oz/115 g

FAT		
	◯ 1 tbsp	◯ 1 tbsp
	◯ 1 tbsp	

LOW-SUGAR VEGGIES		
	◯ ½ cup/50 g	◯ ½ cup/50 g
	◯ ½ cup/50 g	◯ ½ cup/50 g
	◯ ½ cup/50 g	◯ ½ cup/50 g

COMPLEX CARBS		
	◯ ½ cup/50 g	◯ ½ cup/50 g

LOW-SUGAR FRUITS		
	◯ ½ cup/50 g	◯ ½ cup/50 g
	◯ ½ cup/50 g	◯ ½ cup/50 g

CHECK IN

Did you feel satisfied after each meal?

Did you have cravings today?

What's one thing you were grateful for today?

Today's Date:

EXERCISE

LUNCH

BREAKFAST

SNACK

SNACK

DINNER

DAILY NEEDS

WATER		
○ 8 oz/240 ml	○ 8 oz/240 ml
○ 8 oz/240 ml	○ 8 oz/240 ml
○ 8 oz/240 ml	○ 8 oz/240 ml
○ 8 oz/240 ml	○ 8 oz/240 ml
○ 8 oz/240 ml	○ 8 oz/240 ml

PROTEIN	
○ 4 oz/115 g	○ 4 oz/115 g
○ 4 oz/115 g	○ 4 oz/115 g

FAT	
○ 1 tbsp	○ 1 tbsp
○ 1 tbsp	

LOW-SUGAR VEGGIES	
○ ½ cup/50 g	○ ½ cup/50 g
○ ½ cup/50 g	○ ½ cup/50 g
○ ½ cup/50 g	○ ½ cup/50 g

COMPLEX CARBS	
○ ½ cup/50 g	○ ½ cup/50 g

LOW-SUGAR FRUITS	
○ ½ cup/50 g	○ ½ cup/50 g
○ ½ cup/50 g	○ ½ cup/50 g

CHECK IN

Did you feel satisfied after each meal?

Did you have cravings today?

What's one thing you were grateful for today?

Today's Date:

EXERCISE

LUNCH

BREAKFAST

SNACK

SNACK

DINNER

SPLURGE

DAILY NEEDS

WATER		
◯ 8 oz/240 ml	◯ 8 oz/240 ml	
◯ 8 oz/240 ml	◯ 8 oz/240 ml	
◯ 8 oz/240 ml	◯ 8 oz/240 ml	
◯ 8 oz/240 ml	◯ 8 oz/240 ml	
◯ 8 oz/240 ml	◯ 8 oz/240 ml	

PROTEIN
◯ 4 oz/115 g   ◯ 4 oz/115 g
◯ 4 oz/115 g   ◯ 4 oz/115 g

FAT
◯ 1 tbsp   ◯ 1 tbsp
◯ 1 tbsp

LOW-SUGAR VEGGIES
◯ ½ cup/50 g   ◯ ½ cup/50 g
◯ ½ cup/50 g   ◯ ½ cup/50 g
◯ ½ cup/50 g   ◯ ½ cup/50 g

COMPLEX CARBS
◯ ½ cup/50 g   ◯ ½ cup/50 g

LOW-SUGAR FRUITS
◯ ½ cup/50 g   ◯ ½ cup/50 g
◯ ½ cup/50 g   ◯ ½ cup/50 g

CHECK IN

Did you feel satisfied after each meal?

Did you have cravings today?

What's one thing you were grateful for today?

Today's Date:

FOOD AND FITNESS LOG

EXERCISE

LUNCH

BREAKFAST

SNACK

SNACK

DINNER

DAILY NEEDS

WATER
- ( ) 8 oz/240 ml
- ( ) 8 oz/240 ml
- ( ) 8 oz/240 ml
- ( ) 8 oz/240 ml
- ( ) 8 oz/240 ml
- ( ) 8 oz/240 ml
- ( ) 8 oz/240 ml
- ( ) 8 oz/240 ml
- ( ) 8 oz/240 ml
- ( ) 8 oz/240 ml

PROTEIN
- ( ) 4 oz/115 g
- ( ) 4 oz/115 g
- ( ) 4 oz/115 g
- ( ) 4 oz/115 g

FAT
- ( ) 1 tbsp
- ( ) 1 tbsp
- ( ) 1 tbsp

LOW-SUGAR VEGGIES
- ( ) ½ cup/50 g
- ( ) ½ cup/50 g
- ( ) ½ cup/50 g
- ( ) ½ cup/50 g
- ( ) ½ cup/50 g
- ( ) ½ cup/50 g

COMPLEX CARBS
- ( ) ½ cup/50 g
- ( ) ½ cup/50 g

LOW-SUGAR FRUITS
- ( ) ½ cup/50 g
- ( ) ½ cup/50 g
- ( ) ½ cup/50 g
- ( ) ½ cup/50 g

CHECK IN

Did you feel satisfied after each meal?

Did you have cravings today?

What's one thing you were grateful for today?

Today's Date:

EXERCISE

LUNCH

BREAKFAST

SNACK

SNACK

DINNER

DAILY NEEDS

WATER
- ◯ 8 oz/240 ml
- ◯ 8 oz/240 ml
- ◯ 8 oz/240 ml
- ◯ 8 oz/240 ml
- ◯ 8 oz/240 ml

- ◯ 8 oz/240 ml
- ◯ 8 oz/240 ml
- ◯ 8 oz/240 ml
- ◯ 8 oz/240 ml
- ◯ 8 oz/240 ml

PROTEIN
- ◯ 4 oz/115 g
- ◯ 4 oz/115 g

- ◯ 4 oz/115 g
- ◯ 4 oz/115 g

FAT
- ◯ 1 tbsp
- ◯ 1 tbsp

- ◯ 1 tbsp

LOW-SUGAR VEGGIES
- ◯ ½ cup/50 g
- ◯ ½ cup/50 g
- ◯ ½ cup/50 g

- ◯ ½ cup/50 g
- ◯ ½ cup/50 g
- ◯ ½ cup/50 g

COMPLEX CARBS
- ◯ ½ cup/50 g

- ◯ ½ cup/50 g

LOW-SUGAR FRUITS
- ◯ ½ cup/50 g
- ◯ ½ cup/50 g

- ◯ ½ cup/50 g
- ◯ ½ cup/50 g

CHECK IN

Did you feel satisfied after each meal?

Did you have cravings today?

What's one thing you were grateful for today?

Today's Date:

EXERCISE

LUNCH

BREAKFAST

SNACK

SNACK

DINNER

DAILY NEEDS

WATER
- ◯ 8 oz/240 ml ◯ 8 oz/240 ml
- ◯ 8 oz/240 ml ◯ 8 oz/240 ml
- ◯ 8 oz/240 ml ◯ 8 oz/240 ml
- ◯ 8 oz/240 ml ◯ 8 oz/240 ml
- ◯ 8 oz/240 ml ◯ 8 oz/240 ml

PROTEIN
- ◯ 4 oz/115 g ◯ 4 oz/115 g
- ◯ 4 oz/115 g ◯ 4 oz/115 g

FAT
- ◯ 1 tbsp ◯ 1 tbsp
- ◯ 1 tbsp

LOW-SUGAR VEGGIES
- ◯ ½ cup/50 g ◯ ½ cup/50 g
- ◯ ½ cup/50 g ◯ ½ cup/50 g
- ◯ ½ cup/50 g ◯ ½ cup/50 g

COMPLEX CARBS
- ◯ ½ cup/50 g ◯ ½ cup/50 g

LOW-SUGAR FRUITS
- ◯ ½ cup/50 g ◯ ½ cup/50 g
- ◯ ½ cup/50 g ◯ ½ cup/50 g

CHECK IN

Did you feel satisfied after each meal?

Did you have cravings today?

What's one thing you were grateful for today?

Today's Date:

EXERCISE

LUNCH

BREAKFAST

SNACK

SNACK

DINNER

DAILY NEEDS

WATER
- ◯ 8 oz/240 ml
- ◯ 8 oz/240 ml
- ◯ 8 oz/240 ml
- ◯ 8 oz/240 ml
- ◯ 8 oz/240 ml
- ◯ 8 oz/240 ml
- ◯ 8 oz/240 ml
- ◯ 8 oz/240 ml
- ◯ 8 oz/240 ml
- ◯ 8 oz/240 ml

PROTEIN
- ◯ 4 oz/115 g
- ◯ 4 oz/115 g
- ◯ 4 oz/115 g
- ◯ 4 oz/115 g

FAT
- ◯ 1 tbsp
- ◯ 1 tbsp
- ◯ 1 tbsp

LOW-SUGAR VEGGIES
- ◯ ½ cup/50 g
- ◯ ½ cup/50 g
- ◯ ½ cup/50 g
- ◯ ½ cup/50 g
- ◯ ½ cup/50 g
- ◯ ½ cup/50 g

COMPLEX CARBS
- ◯ ½ cup/50 g
- ◯ ½ cup/50 g

LOW-SUGAR FRUITS
- ◯ ½ cup/50 g
- ◯ ½ cup/50 g
- ◯ ½ cup/50 g
- ◯ ½ cup/50 g

CHECK IN

Did you feel satisfied after each meal?

Did you have cravings today?

What's one thing you were grateful for today?

Today's Date:

FOOD AND FITNESS LOG

EXERCISE

LUNCH

BREAKFAST

SNACK

SNACK

DINNER

DAILY NEEDS

WATER		
○ 8 oz/240 ml	○ 8 oz/240 ml	
○ 8 oz/240 ml	○ 8 oz/240 ml	
○ 8 oz/240 ml	○ 8 oz/240 ml	
○ 8 oz/240 ml	○ 8 oz/240 ml	
○ 8 oz/240 ml	○ 8 oz/240 ml	

PROTEIN	
○ 4 oz/115 g	○ 4 oz/115 g
○ 4 oz/115 g	○ 4 oz/115 g

FAT	
○ 1 tbsp	○ 1 tbsp
○ 1 tbsp	

LOW-SUGAR VEGGIES	
○ ½ cup/50 g	○ ½ cup/50 g
○ ½ cup/50 g	○ ½ cup/50 g
○ ½ cup/50 g	○ ½ cup/50 g

COMPLEX CARBS	
○ ½ cup/50 g	○ ½ cup/50 g

LOW-SUGAR FRUITS	
○ ½ cup/50 g	○ ½ cup/50 g
○ ½ cup/50 g	○ ½ cup/50 g

CHECK IN

Did you feel satisfied after each meal?

Did you have cravings today?

What's one thing you were grateful for today?

Today's Date:

FOOD AND FITNESS LOG

EXERCISE

LUNCH

BREAKFAST

SNACK

SNACK

DINNER

DAILY NEEDS

WATER
- ◯ 8 oz/240 ml   ◯ 8 oz/240 ml
- ◯ 8 oz/240 ml   ◯ 8 oz/240 ml
- ◯ 8 oz/240 ml   ◯ 8 oz/240 ml
- ◯ 8 oz/240 ml   ◯ 8 oz/240 ml
- ◯ 8 oz/240 ml   ◯ 8 oz/240 ml

PROTEIN
- ◯ 4 oz/115 g   ◯ 4 oz/115 g
- ◯ 4 oz/115 g   ◯ 4 oz/115 g

FAT
- ◯ 1 tbsp   ◯ 1 tbsp
- ◯ 1 tbsp

LOW-SUGAR VEGGIES
- ◯ ½ cup/50 g   ◯ ½ cup/50 g
- ◯ ½ cup/50 g   ◯ ½ cup/50 g
- ◯ ½ cup/50 g   ◯ ½ cup/50 g

COMPLEX CARBS
- ◯ ½ cup/50 g   ◯ ½ cup/50 g

LOW-SUGAR FRUITS
- ◯ ½ cup/50 g   ◯ ½ cup/50 g
- ◯ ½ cup/50 g   ◯ ½ cup/50 g

CHECK IN

Did you feel satisfied after each meal?

Did you have cravings today?

What's one thing you were grateful for today?

Today's Date:

EXERCISE

LUNCH

BREAKFAST

SNACK

SNACK

DINNER

SPLURGE

DAILY NEEDS

WATER	
○ 8 oz/240 ml	○ 8 oz/240 ml
○ 8 oz/240 ml	○ 8 oz/240 ml
○ 8 oz/240 ml	○ 8 oz/240 ml
○ 8 oz/240 ml	○ 8 oz/240 ml
○ 8 oz/240 ml	○ 8 oz/240 ml

PROTEIN
○ 4 oz/115 g   ○ 4 oz/115 g
○ 4 oz/115 g   ○ 4 oz/115 g

FAT
○ 1 tbsp   ○ 1 tbsp
○ 1 tbsp

LOW-SUGAR VEGGIES
○ ½ cup/50 g   ○ ½ cup/50 g
○ ½ cup/50 g   ○ ½ cup/50 g
○ ½ cup/50 g   ○ ½ cup/50 g

COMPLEX CARBS
○ ½ cup/50 g   ○ ½ cup/50 g

LOW-SUGAR FRUITS
○ ½ cup/50 g   ○ ½ cup/50 g
○ ½ cup/50 g   ○ ½ cup/50 g

CHECK IN

Did you feel satisfied after each meal?

Did you have cravings today?

What's one thing you were grateful for today?

Today's Date:

EXERCISE

LUNCH

BREAKFAST

SNACK

SNACK

DINNER

DAILY NEEDS

WATER		
○ 8 oz/240 ml	○ 8 oz/240 ml
○ 8 oz/240 ml	○ 8 oz/240 ml
○ 8 oz/240 ml	○ 8 oz/240 ml
○ 8 oz/240 ml	○ 8 oz/240 ml
○ 8 oz/240 ml	○ 8 oz/240 ml

PROTEIN		
○ 4 oz/115 g	○ 4 oz/115 g
○ 4 oz/115 g	○ 4 oz/115 g

FAT		
○ 1 tbsp	○ 1 tbsp
○ 1 tbsp	

LOW-SUGAR VEGGIES
○ ½ cup/50 g   ○ ½ cup/50 g
○ ½ cup/50 g   ○ ½ cup/50 g
○ ½ cup/50 g   ○ ½ cup/50 g

COMPLEX CARBS
○ ½ cup/50 g   ○ ½ cup/50 g

LOW-SUGAR FRUITS
○ ½ cup/50 g   ○ ½ cup/50 g
○ ½ cup/50 g   ○ ½ cup/50 g

CHECK IN

Did you feel satisfied after each meal?

Did you have cravings today?

What's one thing you were grateful for today?

Today's Date:

EXERCISE

LUNCH

BREAKFAST

SNACK

SNACK

DINNER

DAILY NEEDS

WATER
- ◯ 8 oz/240 ml
- ◯ 8 oz/240 ml
- ◯ 8 oz/240 ml
- ◯ 8 oz/240 ml
- ◯ 8 oz/240 ml
- ◯ 8 oz/240 ml
- ◯ 8 oz/240 ml
- ◯ 8 oz/240 ml
- ◯ 8 oz/240 ml
- ◯ 8 oz/240 ml

PROTEIN
- ◯ 4 oz/115 g
- ◯ 4 oz/115 g
- ◯ 4 oz/115 g
- ◯ 4 oz/115 g

FAT
- ◯ 1 tbsp
- ◯ 1 tbsp
- ◯ 1 tbsp

LOW-SUGAR VEGGIES
- ◯ ½ cup/50 g
- ◯ ½ cup/50 g
- ◯ ½ cup/50 g
- ◯ ½ cup/50 g
- ◯ ½ cup/50 g
- ◯ ½ cup/50 g

COMPLEX CARBS
- ◯ ½ cup/50 g
- ◯ ½ cup/50 g

LOW-SUGAR FRUITS
- ◯ ½ cup/50 g
- ◯ ½ cup/50 g
- ◯ ½ cup/50 g
- ◯ ½ cup/50 g

CHECK IN

Did you feel satisfied after each meal?

Did you have cravings today?

What's one thing you were grateful for today?

Today's Date:

EXERCISE

LUNCH

BREAKFAST

SNACK

SNACK

DINNER

DAILY NEEDS

WATER
- ◯ 8 oz/240 ml
- ◯ 8 oz/240 ml
- ◯ 8 oz/240 ml
- ◯ 8 oz/240 ml
- ◯ 8 oz/240 ml

- ◯ 8 oz/240 ml
- ◯ 8 oz/240 ml
- ◯ 8 oz/240 ml
- ◯ 8 oz/240 ml
- ◯ 8 oz/240 ml

PROTEIN
- ◯ 4 oz/115 g
- ◯ 4 oz/115 g

- ◯ 4 oz/115 g
- ◯ 4 oz/115 g

FAT
- ◯ 1 tbsp
- ◯ 1 tbsp

- ◯ 1 tbsp

LOW-SUGAR VEGGIES
- ◯ ½ cup/50 g
- ◯ ½ cup/50 g
- ◯ ½ cup/50 g

- ◯ ½ cup/50 g
- ◯ ½ cup/50 g
- ◯ ½ cup/50 g

COMPLEX CARBS
- ◯ ½ cup/50 g

- ◯ ½ cup/50 g

LOW-SUGAR FRUITS
- ◯ ½ cup/50 g
- ◯ ½ cup/50 g

- ◯ ½ cup/50 g
- ◯ ½ cup/50 g

CHECK IN

Did you feel satisfied after each meal?

Did you have cravings today?

What's one thing you were grateful for today?

Today's Date:

FOOD AND FITNESS LOG

EXERCISE

LUNCH

BREAKFAST

SNACK

SNACK

DINNER

DAILY NEEDS

WATER		
◯ 8 oz/240 ml	◯ 8 oz/240 ml	
◯ 8 oz/240 ml	◯ 8 oz/240 ml	
◯ 8 oz/240 ml	◯ 8 oz/240 ml	
◯ 8 oz/240 ml	◯ 8 oz/240 ml	
◯ 8 oz/240 ml	◯ 8 oz/240 ml	

PROTEIN
◯ 4 oz/115 g   ◯ 4 oz/115 g
◯ 4 oz/115 g   ◯ 4 oz/115 g

FAT
◯ 1 tbsp   ◯ 1 tbsp
◯ 1 tbsp

LOW-SUGAR VEGGIES
◯ ½ cup/50 g   ◯ ½ cup/50 g
◯ ½ cup/50 g   ◯ ½ cup/50 g
◯ ½ cup/50 g   ◯ ½ cup/50 g

COMPLEX CARBS
◯ ½ cup/50 g   ◯ ½ cup/50 g

LOW-SUGAR FRUITS
◯ ½ cup/50 g   ◯ ½ cup/50 g
◯ ½ cup/50 g   ◯ ½ cup/50 g

CHECK IN

Did you feel satisfied after each meal?

Did you have cravings today?

What's one thing you were grateful for today?

Today's Date:

FOOD AND FITNESS LOG

EXERCISE

LUNCH

BREAKFAST

SNACK

SNACK

DINNER

DAILY NEEDS

WATER
- ◯ 8 oz/240 ml
- ◯ 8 oz/240 ml
- ◯ 8 oz/240 ml
- ◯ 8 oz/240 ml
- ◯ 8 oz/240 ml
- ◯ 8 oz/240 ml
- ◯ 8 oz/240 ml
- ◯ 8 oz/240 ml
- ◯ 8 oz/240 ml
- ◯ 8 oz/240 ml

PROTEIN
- ◯ 4 oz/115 g
- ◯ 4 oz/115 g
- ◯ 4 oz/115 g
- ◯ 4 oz/115 g

FAT
- ◯ 1 tbsp
- ◯ 1 tbsp
- ◯ 1 tbsp

LOW-SUGAR VEGGIES
- ◯ ½ cup/50 g
- ◯ ½ cup/50 g
- ◯ ½ cup/50 g
- ◯ ½ cup/50 g
- ◯ ½ cup/50 g
- ◯ ½ cup/50 g

COMPLEX CARBS
- ◯ ½ cup/50 g
- ◯ ½ cup/50 g

LOW-SUGAR FRUITS
- ◯ ½ cup/50 g
- ◯ ½ cup/50 g
- ◯ ½ cup/50 g
- ◯ ½ cup/50 g

CHECK IN

Did you feel satisfied after each meal?

Did you have cravings today?

What's one thing you were grateful for today?

Today's Date:

EXERCISE   LUNCH

_____   _____

BREAKFAST   SNACK

_____   _____

SNACK   DINNER

DAILY NEEDS

WATER
- ◯ 8 oz/240 ml   ◯ 8 oz/240 ml
- ◯ 8 oz/240 ml   ◯ 8 oz/240 ml
- ◯ 8 oz/240 ml   ◯ 8 oz/240 ml
- ◯ 8 oz/240 ml   ◯ 8 oz/240 ml
- ◯ 8 oz/240 ml   ◯ 8 oz/240 ml

PROTEIN
- ◯ 4 oz/115 g   ◯ 4 oz/115 g
- ◯ 4 oz/115 g   ◯ 4 oz/115 g

FAT
- ◯ 1 tbsp   ◯ 1 tbsp
- ◯ 1 tbsp

LOW-SUGAR VEGGIES
- ◯ ½ cup/50 g   ◯ ½ cup/50 g
- ◯ ½ cup/50 g   ◯ ½ cup/50 g
- ◯ ½ cup/50 g   ◯ ½ cup/50 g

COMPLEX CARBS
- ◯ ½ cup/50 g   ◯ ½ cup/50 g

LOW-SUGAR FRUITS
- ◯ ½ cup/50 g   ◯ ½ cup/50 g
- ◯ ½ cup/50 g   ◯ ½ cup/50 g

CHECK IN

Did you feel satisfied after each meal?

_____

Did you have cravings today?

_____

What's one thing you were grateful for today?

_____

Today's Date:

FOOD AND FITNESS LOG

EXERCISE

LUNCH

BREAKFAST

SNACK

SNACK

DINNER

SPLURGE

DAILY NEEDS

WATER			LOW-SUGAR VEGGIES		
○ 8 oz/240 ml	○ 8 oz/240 ml		○ ½ cup/50 g	○ ½ cup/50 g
○ 8 oz/240 ml	○ 8 oz/240 ml		○ ½ cup/50 g	○ ½ cup/50 g
○ 8 oz/240 ml	○ 8 oz/240 ml		○ ½ cup/50 g	○ ½ cup/50 g
○ 8 oz/240 ml	○ 8 oz/240 ml			
○ 8 oz/240 ml	○ 8 oz/240 ml			

COMPLEX CARBS ○ ½ cup/50 g   ○ ½ cup/50 g

PROTEIN
○ 4 oz/115 g   ○ 4 oz/115 g
○ 4 oz/115 g   ○ 4 oz/115 g

LOW-SUGAR FRUITS
○ ½ cup/50 g   ○ ½ cup/50 g
○ ½ cup/50 g   ○ ½ cup/50 g

FAT
○ 1 tbsp   ○ 1 tbsp
○ 1 tbsp

CHECK IN

Did you feel satisfied after each meal?

Did you have cravings today?

What's one thing you were grateful for today?

Today's Date:

FOOD AND FITNESS LOG

EXERCISE

LUNCH

BREAKFAST

SNACK

SNACK

DINNER

DAILY NEEDS

WATER
- ◯ 8 oz/240 ml ◯ 8 oz/240 ml
- ◯ 8 oz/240 ml ◯ 8 oz/240 ml
- ◯ 8 oz/240 ml ◯ 8 oz/240 ml
- ◯ 8 oz/240 ml ◯ 8 oz/240 ml
- ◯ 8 oz/240 ml ◯ 8 oz/240 ml

PROTEIN
- ◯ 4 oz/115 g ◯ 4 oz/115 g
- ◯ 4 oz/115 g ◯ 4 oz/115 g

FAT
- ◯ 1 tbsp ◯ 1 tbsp
- ◯ 1 tbsp

LOW-SUGAR VEGGIES
- ◯ ½ cup/50 g ◯ ½ cup/50 g
- ◯ ½ cup/50 g ◯ ½ cup/50 g
- ◯ ½ cup/50 g ◯ ½ cup/50 g

COMPLEX CARBS
- ◯ ½ cup/50 g ◯ ½ cup/50 g

LOW-SUGAR FRUITS
- ◯ ½ cup/50 g ◯ ½ cup/50 g
- ◯ ½ cup/50 g ◯ ½ cup/50 g

CHECK IN

Did you feel satisfied after each meal?

Did you have cravings today?

What's one thing you were grateful for today?

Today's Date:

FOOD AND FITNESS LOG

EXERCISE

LUNCH

BREAKFAST

SNACK

SNACK

DINNER

DAILY NEEDS

WATER

- ◯ 8 oz/240 ml
- ◯ 8 oz/240 ml
- ◯ 8 oz/240 ml
- ◯ 8 oz/240 ml
- ◯ 8 oz/240 ml

- ◯ 8 oz/240 ml
- ◯ 8 oz/240 ml
- ◯ 8 oz/240 ml
- ◯ 8 oz/240 ml
- ◯ 8 oz/240 ml

PROTEIN

- ◯ 4 oz/115 g
- ◯ 4 oz/115 g

- ◯ 4 oz/115 g
- ◯ 4 oz/115 g

FAT

- ◯ 1 tbsp
- ◯ 1 tbsp

- ◯ 1 tbsp

LOW-SUGAR VEGGIES

- ◯ ½ cup/50 g
- ◯ ½ cup/50 g
- ◯ ½ cup/50 g

- ◯ ½ cup/50 g
- ◯ ½ cup/50 g
- ◯ ½ cup/50 g

COMPLEX CARBS

- ◯ ½ cup/50 g

- ◯ ½ cup/50 g

LOW-SUGAR FRUITS

- ◯ ½ cup/50 g
- ◯ ½ cup/50 g

- ◯ ½ cup/50 g
- ◯ ½ cup/50 g

CHECK IN

Did you feel satisfied after each meal?

Did you have cravings today?

What's one thing you were grateful for today?

Today's Date:

FOOD AND FITNESS LOG

EXERCISE

LUNCH

BREAKFAST

SNACK

SNACK

DINNER

DAILY NEEDS

WATER
- ◯ 8 oz/240 ml
- ◯ 8 oz/240 ml
- ◯ 8 oz/240 ml
- ◯ 8 oz/240 ml
- ◯ 8 oz/240 ml
- ◯ 8 oz/240 ml
- ◯ 8 oz/240 ml
- ◯ 8 oz/240 ml
- ◯ 8 oz/240 ml
- ◯ 8 oz/240 ml

PROTEIN
- ◯ 4 oz/115 g
- ◯ 4 oz/115 g
- ◯ 4 oz/115 g
- ◯ 4 oz/115 g

FAT
- ◯ 1 tbsp
- ◯ 1 tbsp
- ◯ 1 tbsp

LOW-SUGAR VEGGIES
- ◯ ½ cup/50 g
- ◯ ½ cup/50 g
- ◯ ½ cup/50 g
- ◯ ½ cup/50 g
- ◯ ½ cup/50 g
- ◯ ½ cup/50 g

COMPLEX CARBS
- ◯ ½ cup/50 g
- ◯ ½ cup/50 g

LOW-SUGAR FRUITS
- ◯ ½ cup/50 g
- ◯ ½ cup/50 g
- ◯ ½ cup/50 g
- ◯ ½ cup/50 g

CHECK IN

Did you feel satisfied after each meal?

Did you have cravings today?

What's one thing you were grateful for today?

Today's Date:

FOOD AND FITNESS LOG

EXERCISE

LUNCH

BREAKFAST

SNACK

SNACK

DINNER

DAILY NEEDS

WATER			LOW-SUGAR VEGGIES		
◯ 8 oz/240 ml	◯ 8 oz/240 ml		◯ ½ cup/50 g	◯ ½ cup/50 g
◯ 8 oz/240 ml	◯ 8 oz/240 ml		◯ ½ cup/50 g	◯ ½ cup/50 g
◯ 8 oz/240 ml	◯ 8 oz/240 ml		◯ ½ cup/50 g	◯ ½ cup/50 g
◯ 8 oz/240 ml	◯ 8 oz/240 ml			
◯ 8 oz/240 ml	◯ 8 oz/240 ml			

COMPLEX CARBS ◯ ½ cup/50 g   ◯ ½ cup/50 g

PROTEIN
◯ 4 oz/115 g   ◯ 4 oz/115 g
◯ 4 oz/115 g   ◯ 4 oz/115 g

LOW-SUGAR FRUITS
◯ ½ cup/50 g   ◯ ½ cup/50 g
◯ ½ cup/50 g   ◯ ½ cup/50 g

FAT
◯ 1 tbsp   ◯ 1 tbsp
◯ 1 tbsp

CHECK IN

Did you feel satisfied after each meal?

Did you have cravings today?

What's one thing you were grateful for today?

Today's Date:

EXERCISE

LUNCH

BREAKFAST

SNACK

SNACK

DINNER

DAILY NEEDS

WATER		
○ 8 oz/240 ml	○ 8 oz/240 ml	
○ 8 oz/240 ml	○ 8 oz/240 ml	
○ 8 oz/240 ml	○ 8 oz/240 ml	
○ 8 oz/240 ml	○ 8 oz/240 ml	
○ 8 oz/240 ml	○ 8 oz/240 ml	

PROTEIN	
○ 4 oz/115 g	○ 4 oz/115 g
○ 4 oz/115 g	○ 4 oz/115 g

FAT	
○ 1 tbsp	○ 1 tbsp
○ 1 tbsp	

LOW-SUGAR VEGGIES	
○ ½ cup/50 g	○ ½ cup/50 g
○ ½ cup/50 g	○ ½ cup/50 g
○ ½ cup/50 g	○ ½ cup/50 g

COMPLEX CARBS	
○ ½ cup/50 g	○ ½ cup/50 g

LOW-SUGAR FRUITS	
○ ½ cup/50 g	○ ½ cup/50 g
○ ½ cup/50 g	○ ½ cup/50 g

CHECK IN

Did you feel satisfied after each meal?

Did you have cravings today?

What's one thing you were grateful for today?

Today's Date:

FOOD AND FITNESS LOG

EXERCISE

LUNCH

BREAKFAST

SNACK

SNACK

DINNER

DAILY NEEDS

WATER
- ◯ 8 oz/240 ml
- ◯ 8 oz/240 ml
- ◯ 8 oz/240 ml
- ◯ 8 oz/240 ml
- ◯ 8 oz/240 ml

- ◯ 8 oz/240 ml
- ◯ 8 oz/240 ml
- ◯ 8 oz/240 ml
- ◯ 8 oz/240 ml
- ◯ 8 oz/240 ml

PROTEIN
- ◯ 4 oz/115 g
- ◯ 4 oz/115 g

- ◯ 4 oz/115 g
- ◯ 4 oz/115 g

FAT
- ◯ 1 tbsp
- ◯ 1 tbsp

- ◯ 1 tbsp

LOW-SUGAR VEGGIES
- ◯ ½ cup/50 g
- ◯ ½ cup/50 g
- ◯ ½ cup/50 g

- ◯ ½ cup/50 g
- ◯ ½ cup/50 g
- ◯ ½ cup/50 g

COMPLEX CARBS
- ◯ ½ cup/50 g

- ◯ ½ cup/50 g

LOW-SUGAR FRUITS
- ◯ ½ cup/50 g
- ◯ ½ cup/50 g

- ◯ ½ cup/50 g
- ◯ ½ cup/50 g

CHECK IN

Did you feel satisfied after each meal?

Did you have cravings today?

What's one thing you were grateful for today?

Today's Date:

EXERCISE

LUNCH

BREAKFAST

SNACK

SNACK

DINNER

SPLURGE

DAILY NEEDS

WATER

- ( ) 8 oz/240 ml
- ( ) 8 oz/240 ml
- ( ) 8 oz/240 ml
- ( ) 8 oz/240 ml
- ( ) 8 oz/240 ml

- ( ) 8 oz/240 ml
- ( ) 8 oz/240 ml
- ( ) 8 oz/240 ml
- ( ) 8 oz/240 ml
- ( ) 8 oz/240 ml

PROTEIN

- ( ) 4 oz/115 g
- ( ) 4 oz/115 g

- ( ) 4 oz/115 g
- ( ) 4 oz/115 g

FAT

- ( ) 1 tbsp
- ( ) 1 tbsp

- ( ) 1 tbsp

LOW-SUGAR VEGGIES

- ( ) ½ cup/50 g
- ( ) ½ cup/50 g
- ( ) ½ cup/50 g

- ( ) ½ cup/50 g
- ( ) ½ cup/50 g
- ( ) ½ cup/50 g

COMPLEX CARBS

- ( ) ½ cup/50 g

- ( ) ½ cup/50 g

LOW-SUGAR FRUITS

- ( ) ½ cup/50 g
- ( ) ½ cup/50 g

- ( ) ½ cup/50 g
- ( ) ½ cup/50 g

CHECK IN

Did you feel satisfied after each meal?

Did you have cravings today?

What's one thing you were grateful for today?

Today's Date:

EXERCISE

LUNCH

BREAKFAST

SNACK

SNACK

DINNER

DAILY NEEDS

WATER

○ 8 oz/240 ml   ○ 8 oz/240 ml
○ 8 oz/240 ml   ○ 8 oz/240 ml
○ 8 oz/240 ml   ○ 8 oz/240 ml
○ 8 oz/240 ml   ○ 8 oz/240 ml
○ 8 oz/240 ml   ○ 8 oz/240 ml

PROTEIN

○ 4 oz/115 g   ○ 4 oz/115 g
○ 4 oz/115 g   ○ 4 oz/115 g

FAT

○ 1 tbsp   ○ 1 tbsp
○ 1 tbsp

LOW-SUGAR VEGGIES

○ ½ cup/50 g   ○ ½ cup/50 g
○ ½ cup/50 g   ○ ½ cup/50 g
○ ½ cup/50 g   ○ ½ cup/50 g

COMPLEX CARBS

○ ½ cup/50 g   ○ ½ cup/50 g

LOW-SUGAR FRUITS

○ ½ cup/50 g   ○ ½ cup/50 g
○ ½ cup/50 g   ○ ½ cup/50 g

CHECK IN

Did you feel satisfied after each meal?

Did you have cravings today?

What's one thing you were grateful for today?

Today's Date:

FOOD AND FITNESS LOG

EXERCISE

LUNCH

BREAKFAST

SNACK

SNACK

DINNER

DAILY NEEDS

WATER		
◯ 8 oz/240 ml	◯ 8 oz/240 ml
◯ 8 oz/240 ml	◯ 8 oz/240 ml
◯ 8 oz/240 ml	◯ 8 oz/240 ml
◯ 8 oz/240 ml	◯ 8 oz/240 ml
◯ 8 oz/240 ml	◯ 8 oz/240 ml

PROTEIN
◯ 4 oz/115 g   ◯ 4 oz/115 g
◯ 4 oz/115 g   ◯ 4 oz/115 g

FAT
◯ 1 tbsp   ◯ 1 tbsp
◯ 1 tbsp

LOW-SUGAR VEGGIES
◯ ½ cup/50 g   ◯ ½ cup/50 g
◯ ½ cup/50 g   ◯ ½ cup/50 g
◯ ½ cup/50 g   ◯ ½ cup/50 g

COMPLEX CARBS
◯ ½ cup/50 g   ◯ ½ cup/50 g

LOW-SUGAR FRUITS
◯ ½ cup/50 g   ◯ ½ cup/50 g
◯ ½ cup/50 g   ◯ ½ cup/50 g

CHECK IN

Did you feel satisfied after each meal?

Did you have cravings today?

What's one thing you were grateful for today?

Today's Date:

FOOD AND FITNESS LOG

EXERCISE

LUNCH

BREAKFAST

SNACK

SNACK

DINNER

DAILY NEEDS

WATER		
○ 8 oz/240 ml	○ 8 oz/240 ml	
○ 8 oz/240 ml	○ 8 oz/240 ml	
○ 8 oz/240 ml	○ 8 oz/240 ml	
○ 8 oz/240 ml	○ 8 oz/240 ml	
○ 8 oz/240 ml	○ 8 oz/240 ml	

PROTEIN	
○ 4 oz/115 g	○ 4 oz/115 g
○ 4 oz/115 g	○ 4 oz/115 g

FAT	
○ 1 tbsp	○ 1 tbsp
○ 1 tbsp	

LOW-SUGAR VEGGIES	
○ ½ cup/50 g	○ ½ cup/50 g
○ ½ cup/50 g	○ ½ cup/50 g
○ ½ cup/50 g	○ ½ cup/50 g

COMPLEX CARBS	
○ ½ cup/50 g	○ ½ cup/50 g

LOW-SUGAR FRUITS	
○ ½ cup/50 g	○ ½ cup/50 g
○ ½ cup/50 g	○ ½ cup/50 g

CHECK IN

Did you feel satisfied after each meal?

Did you have cravings today?

What's one thing you were grateful for today?

Today's Date:

FOOD AND FITNESS LOG

EXERCISE

LUNCH

BREAKFAST

SNACK

SNACK

DINNER

DAILY NEEDS

WATER		
◯ 8 oz/240 ml	◯ 8 oz/240 ml
◯ 8 oz/240 ml	◯ 8 oz/240 ml
◯ 8 oz/240 ml	◯ 8 oz/240 ml
◯ 8 oz/240 ml	◯ 8 oz/240 ml
◯ 8 oz/240 ml	◯ 8 oz/240 ml

PROTEIN
◯ 4 oz/115 g   ◯ 4 oz/115 g
◯ 4 oz/115 g   ◯ 4 oz/115 g

FAT
◯ 1 tbsp   ◯ 1 tbsp
◯ 1 tbsp

LOW-SUGAR VEGGIES
◯ ½ cup/50 g   ◯ ½ cup/50 g
◯ ½ cup/50 g   ◯ ½ cup/50 g
◯ ½ cup/50 g   ◯ ½ cup/50 g

COMPLEX CARBS
◯ ½ cup/50 g   ◯ ½ cup/50 g

LOW-SUGAR FRUITS
◯ ½ cup/50 g   ◯ ½ cup/50 g
◯ ½ cup/50 g   ◯ ½ cup/50 g

CHECK IN

Did you feel satisfied after each meal?

Did you have cravings today?

What's one thing you were grateful for today?

Today's Date:

EXERCISE

LUNCH

BREAKFAST

SNACK

SNACK

DINNER

DAILY NEEDS

WATER
- ◯ 8 oz/240 ml
- ◯ 8 oz/240 ml
- ◯ 8 oz/240 ml
- ◯ 8 oz/240 ml
- ◯ 8 oz/240 ml

- ◯ 8 oz/240 ml
- ◯ 8 oz/240 ml
- ◯ 8 oz/240 ml
- ◯ 8 oz/240 ml
- ◯ 8 oz/240 ml

PROTEIN
- ◯ 4 oz/115 g
- ◯ 4 oz/115 g

- ◯ 4 oz/115 g
- ◯ 4 oz/115 g

FAT
- ◯ 1 tbsp
- ◯ 1 tbsp

- ◯ 1 tbsp

LOW-SUGAR VEGGIES
- ◯ ½ cup/50 g
- ◯ ½ cup/50 g
- ◯ ½ cup/50 g

- ◯ ½ cup/50 g
- ◯ ½ cup/50 g
- ◯ ½ cup/50 g

COMPLEX CARBS
- ◯ ½ cup/50 g

- ◯ ½ cup/50 g

LOW-SUGAR FRUITS
- ◯ ½ cup/50 g
- ◯ ½ cup/50 g

- ◯ ½ cup/50 g
- ◯ ½ cup/50 g

CHECK IN

Did you feel satisfied after each meal?

Did you have cravings today?

What's one thing you were grateful for today?

Today's Date:

EXERCISE

LUNCH

BREAKFAST

SNACK

SNACK

DINNER

DAILY NEEDS

WATER
- ◯ 8 oz/240 ml ◯ 8 oz/240 ml
- ◯ 8 oz/240 ml ◯ 8 oz/240 ml
- ◯ 8 oz/240 ml ◯ 8 oz/240 ml
- ◯ 8 oz/240 ml ◯ 8 oz/240 ml
- ◯ 8 oz/240 ml ◯ 8 oz/240 ml

PROTEIN
- ◯ 4 oz/115 g ◯ 4 oz/115 g
- ◯ 4 oz/115 g ◯ 4 oz/115 g

FAT
- ◯ 1 tbsp ◯ 1 tbsp
- ◯ 1 tbsp

LOW-SUGAR VEGGIES
- ◯ ½ cup/50 g ◯ ½ cup/50 g
- ◯ ½ cup/50 g ◯ ½ cup/50 g
- ◯ ½ cup/50 g ◯ ½ cup/50 g

COMPLEX CARBS
- ◯ ½ cup/50 g ◯ ½ cup/50 g

LOW-SUGAR FRUITS
- ◯ ½ cup/50 g ◯ ½ cup/50 g
- ◯ ½ cup/50 g ◯ ½ cup/50 g

CHECK IN

Did you feel satisfied after each meal?

Did you have cravings today?

What's one thing you were grateful for today?

Today's Date:

EXERCISE

LUNCH

BREAKFAST

SNACK

SNACK

DINNER

SPLURGE

DAILY NEEDS

WATER		
○ 8 oz/240 ml	○ 8 oz/240 ml
○ 8 oz/240 ml	○ 8 oz/240 ml
○ 8 oz/240 ml	○ 8 oz/240 ml
○ 8 oz/240 ml	○ 8 oz/240 ml
○ 8 oz/240 ml	○ 8 oz/240 ml

PROTEIN
○ 4 oz/115 g   ○ 4 oz/115 g
○ 4 oz/115 g   ○ 4 oz/115 g

FAT
○ 1 tbsp   ○ 1 tbsp
○ 1 tbsp

LOW-SUGAR VEGGIES
○ ½ cup/50 g   ○ ½ cup/50 g
○ ½ cup/50 g   ○ ½ cup/50 g
○ ½ cup/50 g   ○ ½ cup/50 g

COMPLEX CARBS
○ ½ cup/50 g   ○ ½ cup/50 g

LOW-SUGAR FRUITS
○ ½ cup/50 g   ○ ½ cup/50 g
○ ½ cup/50 g   ○ ½ cup/50 g

CHECK IN

Did you feel satisfied after each meal?

Did you have cravings today?

What's one thing you were grateful for today?

Today's Date:

FOOD AND FITNESS LOG

EXERCISE

LUNCH

BREAKFAST

SNACK

SNACK

DINNER

DAILY NEEDS

WATER
○ 8 oz/240 ml   ○ 8 oz/240 ml
○ 8 oz/240 ml   ○ 8 oz/240 ml
○ 8 oz/240 ml   ○ 8 oz/240 ml
○ 8 oz/240 ml   ○ 8 oz/240 ml
○ 8 oz/240 ml   ○ 8 oz/240 ml

PROTEIN
○ 4 oz/115 g   ○ 4 oz/115 g
○ 4 oz/115 g   ○ 4 oz/115 g

FAT
○ 1 tbsp   ○ 1 tbsp
○ 1 tbsp

LOW-SUGAR VEGGIES
○ ½ cup/50 g   ○ ½ cup/50 g
○ ½ cup/50 g   ○ ½ cup/50 g
○ ½ cup/50 g   ○ ½ cup/50 g

COMPLEX CARBS
○ ½ cup/50 g   ○ ½ cup/50 g

LOW-SUGAR FRUITS
○ ½ cup/50 g   ○ ½ cup/50 g
○ ½ cup/50 g   ○ ½ cup/50 g

CHECK IN

Did you feel satisfied after each meal?

Did you have cravings today?

What's one thing you were grateful for today?

Today's Date:

EXERCISE

LUNCH

BREAKFAST

SNACK

SNACK

DINNER

DAILY NEEDS

WATER		
◯ 8 oz/240 ml	◯ 8 oz/240 ml
◯ 8 oz/240 ml	◯ 8 oz/240 ml
◯ 8 oz/240 ml	◯ 8 oz/240 ml
◯ 8 oz/240 ml	◯ 8 oz/240 ml
◯ 8 oz/240 ml	◯ 8 oz/240 ml

PROTEIN
◯ 4 oz/115 g   ◯ 4 oz/115 g
◯ 4 oz/115 g   ◯ 4 oz/115 g

FAT
◯ 1 tbsp   ◯ 1 tbsp
◯ 1 tbsp

LOW-SUGAR VEGGIES
◯ ½ cup/50 g   ◯ ½ cup/50 g
◯ ½ cup/50 g   ◯ ½ cup/50 g
◯ ½ cup/50 g   ◯ ½ cup/50 g

COMPLEX CARBS
◯ ½ cup/50 g   ◯ ½ cup/50 g

LOW-SUGAR FRUITS
◯ ½ cup/50 g   ◯ ½ cup/50 g
◯ ½ cup/50 g   ◯ ½ cup/50 g

CHECK IN

Did you feel satisfied after each meal?

Did you have cravings today?

What's one thing you were grateful for today?

Today's Date:

FOOD AND FITNESS LOG

EXERCISE

LUNCH

BREAKFAST

SNACK

SNACK

DINNER

DAILY NEEDS

WATER			LOW-SUGAR VEGGIES		
	○ 8 oz/240 ml	○ 8 oz/240 ml		○ ½ cup/50 g	○ ½ cup/50 g
	○ 8 oz/240 ml	○ 8 oz/240 ml		○ ½ cup/50 g	○ ½ cup/50 g
	○ 8 oz/240 ml	○ 8 oz/240 ml		○ ½ cup/50 g	○ ½ cup/50 g

○ 8 oz/240 ml   ○ 8 oz/240 ml

○ 8 oz/240 ml   ○ 8 oz/240 ml

COMPLEX CARBS ○ ½ cup/50 g   ○ ½ cup/50 g

PROTEIN

○ 4 oz/115 g   ○ 4 oz/115 g

○ 4 oz/115 g   ○ 4 oz/115 g

LOW-SUGAR FRUITS ○ ½ cup/50 g   ○ ½ cup/50 g

○ ½ cup/50 g   ○ ½ cup/50 g

FAT

○ 1 tbsp   ○ 1 tbsp

○ 1 tbsp

CHECK IN

Did you feel satisfied after each meal?

Did you have cravings today?

What's one thing you were grateful for today?

Today's Date:

EXERCISE

LUNCH

BREAKFAST

SNACK

SNACK

DINNER

DAILY NEEDS

WATER		
◯ 8 oz/240 ml	◯ 8 oz/240 ml
◯ 8 oz/240 ml	◯ 8 oz/240 ml
◯ 8 oz/240 ml	◯ 8 oz/240 ml
◯ 8 oz/240 ml	◯ 8 oz/240 ml
◯ 8 oz/240 ml	◯ 8 oz/240 ml

PROTEIN	
◯ 4 oz/115 g	◯ 4 oz/115 g
◯ 4 oz/115 g	◯ 4 oz/115 g

FAT	
◯ 1 tbsp	◯ 1 tbsp
◯ 1 tbsp	

LOW-SUGAR VEGGIES
◯ ½ cup/50 g   ◯ ½ cup/50 g
◯ ½ cup/50 g   ◯ ½ cup/50 g
◯ ½ cup/50 g   ◯ ½ cup/50 g

COMPLEX CARBS
◯ ½ cup/50 g   ◯ ½ cup/50 g

LOW-SUGAR FRUITS
◯ ½ cup/50 g   ◯ ½ cup/50 g
◯ ½ cup/50 g   ◯ ½ cup/50 g

CHECK IN

Did you feel satisfied after each meal?

Did you have cravings today?

What's one thing you were grateful for today?

Today's Date:

FOOD AND FITNESS LOG

EXERCISE

LUNCH

BREAKFAST

SNACK

SNACK

DINNER

DAILY NEEDS

WATER
- ◯ 8 oz/240 ml
- ◯ 8 oz/240 ml
- ◯ 8 oz/240 ml
- ◯ 8 oz/240 ml
- ◯ 8 oz/240 ml

- ◯ 8 oz/240 ml
- ◯ 8 oz/240 ml
- ◯ 8 oz/240 ml
- ◯ 8 oz/240 ml
- ◯ 8 oz/240 ml

PROTEIN
- ◯ 4 oz/115 g
- ◯ 4 oz/115 g

- ◯ 4 oz/115 g
- ◯ 4 oz/115 g

FAT
- ◯ 1 tbsp
- ◯ 1 tbsp

- ◯ 1 tbsp

LOW-SUGAR VEGGIES
- ◯ ½ cup/50 g
- ◯ ½ cup/50 g
- ◯ ½ cup/50 g

- ◯ ½ cup/50 g
- ◯ ½ cup/50 g
- ◯ ½ cup/50 g

COMPLEX CARBS
- ◯ ½ cup/50 g
- ◯ ½ cup/50 g

LOW-SUGAR FRUITS
- ◯ ½ cup/50 g
- ◯ ½ cup/50 g

- ◯ ½ cup/50 g
- ◯ ½ cup/50 g

CHECK IN

Did you feel satisfied after each meal?

Did you have cravings today?

What's one thing you were grateful for today?

Today's Date:

FOOD AND FITNESS LOG

EXERCISE

LUNCH

BREAKFAST

SNACK

SNACK

DINNER

DAILY NEEDS

WATER
- ◯ 8 oz/240 ml
- ◯ 8 oz/240 ml
- ◯ 8 oz/240 ml
- ◯ 8 oz/240 ml
- ◯ 8 oz/240 ml
- ◯ 8 oz/240 ml
- ◯ 8 oz/240 ml
- ◯ 8 oz/240 ml
- ◯ 8 oz/240 ml
- ◯ 8 oz/240 ml

PROTEIN
- ◯ 4 oz/115 g
- ◯ 4 oz/115 g
- ◯ 4 oz/115 g
- ◯ 4 oz/115 g

FAT
- ◯ 1 tbsp
- ◯ 1 tbsp
- ◯ 1 tbsp

LOW-SUGAR VEGGIES
- ◯ ½ cup/50 g
- ◯ ½ cup/50 g
- ◯ ½ cup/50 g
- ◯ ½ cup/50 g
- ◯ ½ cup/50 g
- ◯ ½ cup/50 g

COMPLEX CARBS
- ◯ ½ cup/50 g
- ◯ ½ cup/50 g

LOW-SUGAR FRUITS
- ◯ ½ cup/50 g
- ◯ ½ cup/50 g
- ◯ ½ cup/50 g
- ◯ ½ cup/50 g

CHECK IN

Did you feel satisfied after each meal?

Did you have cravings today?

What's one thing you were grateful for today?

Today's Date:

FOOD AND FITNESS LOG

EXERCISE

LUNCH

BREAKFAST

SNACK

SNACK

DINNER

SPLURGE

DAILY NEEDS

WATER		
◯ 8 oz/240 ml	◯ 8 oz/240 ml	
◯ 8 oz/240 ml	◯ 8 oz/240 ml	
◯ 8 oz/240 ml	◯ 8 oz/240 ml	
◯ 8 oz/240 ml	◯ 8 oz/240 ml	
◯ 8 oz/240 ml	◯ 8 oz/240 ml	

PROTEIN
◯ 4 oz/115 g ◯ 4 oz/115 g
◯ 4 oz/115 g ◯ 4 oz/115 g

FAT
◯ 1 tbsp ◯ 1 tbsp
◯ 1 tbsp

LOW-SUGAR VEGGIES
◯ ½ cup/50 g ◯ ½ cup/50 g
◯ ½ cup/50 g ◯ ½ cup/50 g
◯ ½ cup/50 g ◯ ½ cup/50 g

COMPLEX CARBS
◯ ½ cup/50 g ◯ ½ cup/50 g

LOW-SUGAR FRUITS
◯ ½ cup/50 g ◯ ½ cup/50 g
◯ ½ cup/50 g ◯ ½ cup/50 g

CHECK IN

Did you feel satisfied after each meal?

Did you have cravings today?

What's one thing you were grateful for today?

Today's Date:

EXERCISE

LUNCH

BREAKFAST

SNACK

SNACK

DINNER

DAILY NEEDS

WATER
- ◯ 8 oz/240 ml
- ◯ 8 oz/240 ml
- ◯ 8 oz/240 ml
- ◯ 8 oz/240 ml
- ◯ 8 oz/240 ml

- ◯ 8 oz/240 ml
- ◯ 8 oz/240 ml
- ◯ 8 oz/240 ml
- ◯ 8 oz/240 ml
- ◯ 8 oz/240 ml

PROTEIN
- ◯ 4 oz/115 g
- ◯ 4 oz/115 g

- ◯ 4 oz/115 g
- ◯ 4 oz/115 g

FAT
- ◯ 1 tbsp
- ◯ 1 tbsp

- ◯ 1 tbsp

LOW-SUGAR VEGGIES
- ◯ ½ cup/50 g
- ◯ ½ cup/50 g
- ◯ ½ cup/50 g

- ◯ ½ cup/50 g
- ◯ ½ cup/50 g
- ◯ ½ cup/50 g

COMPLEX CARBS
- ◯ ½ cup/50 g

- ◯ ½ cup/50 g

LOW-SUGAR FRUITS
- ◯ ½ cup/50 g
- ◯ ½ cup/50 g

- ◯ ½ cup/50 g
- ◯ ½ cup/50 g

CHECK IN

Did you feel satisfied after each meal?

Did you have cravings today?

What's one thing you were grateful for today?

Today's Date:

FOOD AND FITNESS LOG

EXERCISE

LUNCH

BREAKFAST

SNACK

SNACK

DINNER

DAILY NEEDS

WATER	◯ 8 oz/240 ml	◯ 8 oz/240 ml	LOW-SUGAR VEGGIES	◯ ½ cup/50 g	◯ ½ cup/50 g
	◯ 8 oz/240 ml	◯ 8 oz/240 ml		◯ ½ cup/50 g	◯ ½ cup/50 g
	◯ 8 oz/240 ml	◯ 8 oz/240 ml		◯ ½ cup/50 g	◯ ½ cup/50 g
	◯ 8 oz/240 ml	◯ 8 oz/240 ml	COMPLEX CARBS	◯ ½ cup/50 g	◯ ½ cup/50 g
	◯ 8 oz/240 ml	◯ 8 oz/240 ml			
PROTEIN	◯ 4 oz/115 g	◯ 4 oz/115 g	LOW-SUGAR FRUITS	◯ ½ cup/50 g	◯ ½ cup/50 g
	◯ 4 oz/115 g	◯ 4 oz/115 g		◯ ½ cup/50 g	◯ ½ cup/50 g
FAT	◯ 1 tbsp	◯ 1 tbsp			
	◯ 1 tbsp				

CHECK IN

Did you feel satisfied after each meal?

Did you have cravings today?

What's one thing you were grateful for today?

Today's Date:

EXERCISE

LUNCH

BREAKFAST

SNACK

SNACK

DINNER

DAILY NEEDS

WATER
- ◯ 8 oz/240 ml
- ◯ 8 oz/240 ml
- ◯ 8 oz/240 ml
- ◯ 8 oz/240 ml
- ◯ 8 oz/240 ml

- ◯ 8 oz/240 ml
- ◯ 8 oz/240 ml
- ◯ 8 oz/240 ml
- ◯ 8 oz/240 ml
- ◯ 8 oz/240 ml

PROTEIN
- ◯ 4 oz/115 g
- ◯ 4 oz/115 g

- ◯ 4 oz/115 g
- ◯ 4 oz/115 g

FAT
- ◯ 1 tbsp
- ◯ 1 tbsp

- ◯ 1 tbsp

LOW-SUGAR VEGGIES
- ◯ ½ cup/50 g
- ◯ ½ cup/50 g
- ◯ ½ cup/50 g

- ◯ ½ cup/50 g
- ◯ ½ cup/50 g
- ◯ ½ cup/50 g

COMPLEX CARBS
- ◯ ½ cup/50 g

- ◯ ½ cup/50 g

LOW-SUGAR FRUITS
- ◯ ½ cup/50 g
- ◯ ½ cup/50 g

- ◯ ½ cup/50 g
- ◯ ½ cup/50 g

CHECK IN

Did you feel satisfied after each meal?

Did you have cravings today?

What's one thing you were grateful for today?

Today's Date:

EXERCISE

LUNCH

BREAKFAST

SNACK

SNACK

DINNER

DAILY NEEDS

WATER
- ◯ 8 oz/240 ml
- ◯ 8 oz/240 ml
- ◯ 8 oz/240 ml
- ◯ 8 oz/240 ml
- ◯ 8 oz/240 ml
- ◯ 8 oz/240 ml
- ◯ 8 oz/240 ml
- ◯ 8 oz/240 ml
- ◯ 8 oz/240 ml
- ◯ 8 oz/240 ml

PROTEIN
- ◯ 4 oz/115 g
- ◯ 4 oz/115 g
- ◯ 4 oz/115 g
- ◯ 4 oz/115 g

FAT
- ◯ 1 tbsp
- ◯ 1 tbsp
- ◯ 1 tbsp

LOW-SUGAR VEGGIES
- ◯ ½ cup/50 g
- ◯ ½ cup/50 g
- ◯ ½ cup/50 g
- ◯ ½ cup/50 g
- ◯ ½ cup/50 g
- ◯ ½ cup/50 g

COMPLEX CARBS
- ◯ ½ cup/50 g
- ◯ ½ cup/50 g

LOW-SUGAR FRUITS
- ◯ ½ cup/50 g
- ◯ ½ cup/50 g
- ◯ ½ cup/50 g
- ◯ ½ cup/50 g

CHECK IN

Did you feel satisfied after each meal?

Did you have cravings today?

What's one thing you were grateful for today?

Today's Date:

EXERCISE

LUNCH

_____

BREAKFAST

SNACK

_____

SNACK

DINNER

DAILY NEEDS

WATER		
○ 8 oz/240 ml	○ 8 oz/240 ml	
○ 8 oz/240 ml	○ 8 oz/240 ml	
○ 8 oz/240 ml	○ 8 oz/240 ml	
○ 8 oz/240 ml	○ 8 oz/240 ml	
○ 8 oz/240 ml	○ 8 oz/240 ml	

PROTEIN	
○ 4 oz/115 g	○ 4 oz/115 g
○ 4 oz/115 g	○ 4 oz/115 g

FAT	
○ 1 tbsp	○ 1 tbsp
○ 1 tbsp	

LOW-SUGAR VEGGIES	
○ ½ cup/50 g	○ ½ cup/50 g
○ ½ cup/50 g	○ ½ cup/50 g
○ ½ cup/50 g	○ ½ cup/50 g

COMPLEX CARBS	
○ ½ cup/50 g	○ ½ cup/50 g

LOW-SUGAR FRUITS	
○ ½ cup/50 g	○ ½ cup/50 g
○ ½ cup/50 g	○ ½ cup/50 g

CHECK IN

Did you feel satisfied after each meal?

_____

Did you have cravings today?

_____

What's one thing you were grateful for today?

_____

Today's Date:

FOOD AND FITNESS LOG

EXERCISE

LUNCH

BREAKFAST

SNACK

SNACK

DINNER

DAILY NEEDS

WATER
- ( ) 8 oz/240 ml
- ( ) 8 oz/240 ml
- ( ) 8 oz/240 ml
- ( ) 8 oz/240 ml
- ( ) 8 oz/240 ml
- ( ) 8 oz/240 ml
- ( ) 8 oz/240 ml
- ( ) 8 oz/240 ml
- ( ) 8 oz/240 ml
- ( ) 8 oz/240 ml

PROTEIN
- ( ) 4 oz/115 g
- ( ) 4 oz/115 g
- ( ) 4 oz/115 g
- ( ) 4 oz/115 g

FAT
- ( ) 1 tbsp
- ( ) 1 tbsp
- ( ) 1 tbsp

LOW-SUGAR VEGGIES
- ( ) ½ cup/50 g
- ( ) ½ cup/50 g
- ( ) ½ cup/50 g
- ( ) ½ cup/50 g
- ( ) ½ cup/50 g
- ( ) ½ cup/50 g

COMPLEX CARBS
- ( ) ½ cup/50 g
- ( ) ½ cup/50 g

LOW-SUGAR FRUITS
- ( ) ½ cup/50 g
- ( ) ½ cup/50 g
- ( ) ½ cup/50 g
- ( ) ½ cup/50 g

CHECK IN

Did you feel satisfied after each meal?

Did you have cravings today?

What's one thing you were grateful for today?

Today's Date:

EXERCISE

LUNCH

BREAKFAST

SNACK

SNACK

DINNER

SPLURGE

DAILY NEEDS

WATER

◯ 8 oz/240 ml   ◯ 8 oz/240 ml
◯ 8 oz/240 ml   ◯ 8 oz/240 ml
◯ 8 oz/240 ml   ◯ 8 oz/240 ml
◯ 8 oz/240 ml   ◯ 8 oz/240 ml
◯ 8 oz/240 ml   ◯ 8 oz/240 ml

PROTEIN

◯ 4 oz/115 g   ◯ 4 oz/115 g
◯ 4 oz/115 g   ◯ 4 oz/115 g

FAT

◯ 1 tbsp   ◯ 1 tbsp
◯ 1 tbsp

LOW-SUGAR VEGGIES

◯ ½ cup/50 g   ◯ ½ cup/50 g
◯ ½ cup/50 g   ◯ ½ cup/50 g
◯ ½ cup/50 g   ◯ ½ cup/50 g

COMPLEX CARBS

◯ ½ cup/50 g   ◯ ½ cup/50 g

LOW-SUGAR FRUITS

◯ ½ cup/50 g   ◯ ½ cup/50 g
◯ ½ cup/50 g   ◯ ½ cup/50 g

CHECK IN

Did you feel satisfied after each meal?

Did you have cravings today?

What's one thing you were grateful for today?

Today's Date:

EXERCISE

LUNCH

BREAKFAST

SNACK

SNACK

DINNER

DAILY NEEDS

WATER

⃝ 8 oz/240 ml	⃝ 8 oz/240 ml
⃝ 8 oz/240 ml	⃝ 8 oz/240 ml
⃝ 8 oz/240 ml	⃝ 8 oz/240 ml
⃝ 8 oz/240 ml	⃝ 8 oz/240 ml
⃝ 8 oz/240 ml	⃝ 8 oz/240 ml

PROTEIN

| ⃝ 4 oz/115 g | ⃝ 4 oz/115 g |
| ⃝ 4 oz/115 g | ⃝ 4 oz/115 g |

FAT

| ⃝ 1 tbsp | ⃝ 1 tbsp |
| ⃝ 1 tbsp | |

LOW-SUGAR VEGGIES

⃝ ½ cup/50 g	⃝ ½ cup/50 g
⃝ ½ cup/50 g	⃝ ½ cup/50 g
⃝ ½ cup/50 g	⃝ ½ cup/50 g

COMPLEX CARBS

| ⃝ ½ cup/50 g | ⃝ ½ cup/50 g |

LOW-SUGAR FRUITS

| ⃝ ½ cup/50 g | ⃝ ½ cup/50 g |
| ⃝ ½ cup/50 g | ⃝ ½ cup/50 g |

CHECK IN

Did you feel satisfied after each meal?

Did you have cravings today?

What's one thing you were grateful for today?

Today's Date:

EXERCISE   LUNCH

_____   _____

BREAKFAST   SNACK

_____   _____

SNACK   DINNER

DAILY NEEDS

WATER
- ◯ 8 oz/240 ml   ◯ 8 oz/240 ml
- ◯ 8 oz/240 ml   ◯ 8 oz/240 ml
- ◯ 8 oz/240 ml   ◯ 8 oz/240 ml
- ◯ 8 oz/240 ml   ◯ 8 oz/240 ml
- ◯ 8 oz/240 ml   ◯ 8 oz/240 ml

PROTEIN
- ◯ 4 oz/115 g   ◯ 4 oz/115 g
- ◯ 4 oz/115 g   ◯ 4 oz/115 g

FAT
- ◯ 1 tbsp   ◯ 1 tbsp
- ◯ 1 tbsp

LOW-SUGAR VEGGIES
- ◯ ½ cup/50 g   ◯ ½ cup/50 g
- ◯ ½ cup/50 g   ◯ ½ cup/50 g
- ◯ ½ cup/50 g   ◯ ½ cup/50 g

COMPLEX CARBS
- ◯ ½ cup/50 g   ◯ ½ cup/50 g

LOW-SUGAR FRUITS
- ◯ ½ cup/50 g   ◯ ½ cup/50 g
- ◯ ½ cup/50 g   ◯ ½ cup/50 g

CHECK IN

Did you feel satisfied after each meal?

_____

Did you have cravings today?

_____

What's one thing you were grateful for today?

_____

Today's Date:

EXERCISE

LUNCH

BREAKFAST

SNACK

SNACK

DINNER

DAILY NEEDS

WATER

- ◯ 8 oz/240 ml
- ◯ 8 oz/240 ml
- ◯ 8 oz/240 ml
- ◯ 8 oz/240 ml
- ◯ 8 oz/240 ml

- ◯ 8 oz/240 ml
- ◯ 8 oz/240 ml
- ◯ 8 oz/240 ml
- ◯ 8 oz/240 ml
- ◯ 8 oz/240 ml

PROTEIN

- ◯ 4 oz/115 g
- ◯ 4 oz/115 g

- ◯ 4 oz/115 g
- ◯ 4 oz/115 g

FAT

- ◯ 1 tbsp
- ◯ 1 tbsp

- ◯ 1 tbsp

LOW-SUGAR VEGGIES

- ◯ ½ cup/50 g
- ◯ ½ cup/50 g
- ◯ ½ cup/50 g

- ◯ ½ cup/50 g
- ◯ ½ cup/50 g
- ◯ ½ cup/50 g

COMPLEX CARBS

- ◯ ½ cup/50 g
- ◯ ½ cup/50 g

LOW-SUGAR FRUITS

- ◯ ½ cup/50 g
- ◯ ½ cup/50 g

- ◯ ½ cup/50 g
- ◯ ½ cup/50 g

CHECK IN

Did you feel satisfied after each meal?

Did you have cravings today?

What's one thing you were grateful for today?

Today's Date:

FOOD AND FITNESS LOG

EXERCISE

LUNCH

BREAKFAST

SNACK

SNACK

DINNER

DAILY NEEDS

WATER			LOW-SUGAR VEGGIES		
◯ 8 oz/240 ml	◯ 8 oz/240 ml		◯ ½ cup/50 g	◯ ½ cup/50 g
◯ 8 oz/240 ml	◯ 8 oz/240 ml		◯ ½ cup/50 g	◯ ½ cup/50 g
◯ 8 oz/240 ml	◯ 8 oz/240 ml		◯ ½ cup/50 g	◯ ½ cup/50 g
◯ 8 oz/240 ml	◯ 8 oz/240 ml			
◯ 8 oz/240 ml	◯ 8 oz/240 ml		COMPLEX CARBS ◯ ½ cup/50 g	◯ ½ cup/50 g

PROTEIN
◯ 4 oz/115 g   ◯ 4 oz/115 g
◯ 4 oz/115 g   ◯ 4 oz/115 g

LOW-SUGAR FRUITS
◯ ½ cup/50 g   ◯ ½ cup/50 g
◯ ½ cup/50 g   ◯ ½ cup/50 g

FAT
◯ 1 tbsp   ◯ 1 tbsp
◯ 1 tbsp

CHECK IN

Did you feel satisfied after each meal?

Did you have cravings today?

What's one thing you were grateful for today?

Today's Date:

EXERCISE

LUNCH

BREAKFAST

SNACK

SNACK

DINNER

DAILY NEEDS

WATER
- ◯ 8 oz/240 ml
- ◯ 8 oz/240 ml
- ◯ 8 oz/240 ml
- ◯ 8 oz/240 ml
- ◯ 8 oz/240 ml

- ◯ 8 oz/240 ml
- ◯ 8 oz/240 ml
- ◯ 8 oz/240 ml
- ◯ 8 oz/240 ml
- ◯ 8 oz/240 ml

PROTEIN
- ◯ 4 oz/115 g
- ◯ 4 oz/115 g

- ◯ 4 oz/115 g
- ◯ 4 oz/115 g

FAT
- ◯ 1 tbsp
- ◯ 1 tbsp

- ◯ 1 tbsp

LOW-SUGAR VEGGIES
- ◯ ½ cup/50 g
- ◯ ½ cup/50 g
- ◯ ½ cup/50 g

- ◯ ½ cup/50 g
- ◯ ½ cup/50 g
- ◯ ½ cup/50 g

COMPLEX CARBS
- ◯ ½ cup/50 g

- ◯ ½ cup/50 g

LOW-SUGAR FRUITS
- ◯ ½ cup/50 g
- ◯ ½ cup/50 g

- ◯ ½ cup/50 g
- ◯ ½ cup/50 g

CHECK IN

Did you feel satisfied after each meal?

Did you have cravings today?

What's one thing you were grateful for today?

Today's Date:

EXERCISE

LUNCH

BREAKFAST

SNACK

SNACK

DINNER

DAILY NEEDS

WATER

- ◯ 8 oz/240 ml
- ◯ 8 oz/240 ml
- ◯ 8 oz/240 ml
- ◯ 8 oz/240 ml
- ◯ 8 oz/240 ml

- ◯ 8 oz/240 ml
- ◯ 8 oz/240 ml
- ◯ 8 oz/240 ml
- ◯ 8 oz/240 ml
- ◯ 8 oz/240 ml

PROTEIN

- ◯ 4 oz/115 g
- ◯ 4 oz/115 g

- ◯ 4 oz/115 g
- ◯ 4 oz/115 g

FAT

- ◯ 1 tbsp
- ◯ 1 tbsp

- ◯ 1 tbsp

LOW-SUGAR VEGGIES

- ◯ ½ cup/50 g
- ◯ ½ cup/50 g
- ◯ ½ cup/50 g

- ◯ ½ cup/50 g
- ◯ ½ cup/50 g
- ◯ ½ cup/50 g

COMPLEX CARBS

- ◯ ½ cup/50 g

- ◯ ½ cup/50 g

LOW-SUGAR FRUITS

- ◯ ½ cup/50 g
- ◯ ½ cup/50 g

- ◯ ½ cup/50 g
- ◯ ½ cup/50 g

CHECK IN

Did you feel satisfied after each meal?

Did you have cravings today?

What's one thing you were grateful for today?

Today's Date:

EXERCISE

LUNCH

BREAKFAST

SNACK

SNACK

DINNER

SPLURGE

DAILY NEEDS

WATER
- ◯ 8 oz/240 ml
- ◯ 8 oz/240 ml
- ◯ 8 oz/240 ml
- ◯ 8 oz/240 ml
- ◯ 8 oz/240 ml

- ◯ 8 oz/240 ml
- ◯ 8 oz/240 ml
- ◯ 8 oz/240 ml
- ◯ 8 oz/240 ml
- ◯ 8 oz/240 ml

PROTEIN
- ◯ 4 oz/115 g
- ◯ 4 oz/115 g

- ◯ 4 oz/115 g
- ◯ 4 oz/115 g

FAT
- ◯ 1 tbsp
- ◯ 1 tbsp

- ◯ 1 tbsp

LOW-SUGAR VEGGIES
- ◯ ½ cup/50 g
- ◯ ½ cup/50 g
- ◯ ½ cup/50 g

- ◯ ½ cup/50 g
- ◯ ½ cup/50 g
- ◯ ½ cup/50 g

COMPLEX CARBS
- ◯ ½ cup/50 g

- ◯ ½ cup/50 g

LOW-SUGAR FRUITS
- ◯ ½ cup/50 g
- ◯ ½ cup/50 g

- ◯ ½ cup/50 g
- ◯ ½ cup/50 g

CHECK IN

Did you feel satisfied after each meal?

Did you have cravings today?

What's one thing you were grateful for today?

Today's Date:

EXERCISE

LUNCH

BREAKFAST

SNACK

SNACK

DINNER

DAILY NEEDS

WATER
- ◯ 8 oz/240 ml
- ◯ 8 oz/240 ml
- ◯ 8 oz/240 ml
- ◯ 8 oz/240 ml
- ◯ 8 oz/240 ml

- ◯ 8 oz/240 ml
- ◯ 8 oz/240 ml
- ◯ 8 oz/240 ml
- ◯ 8 oz/240 ml
- ◯ 8 oz/240 ml

PROTEIN
- ◯ 4 oz/115 g
- ◯ 4 oz/115 g

- ◯ 4 oz/115 g
- ◯ 4 oz/115 g

FAT
- ◯ 1 tbsp
- ◯ 1 tbsp

- ◯ 1 tbsp

LOW-SUGAR VEGGIES
- ◯ ½ cup/50 g
- ◯ ½ cup/50 g
- ◯ ½ cup/50 g

- ◯ ½ cup/50 g
- ◯ ½ cup/50 g
- ◯ ½ cup/50 g

COMPLEX CARBS
- ◯ ½ cup/50 g

- ◯ ½ cup/50 g

LOW-SUGAR FRUITS
- ◯ ½ cup/50 g
- ◯ ½ cup/50 g

- ◯ ½ cup/50 g
- ◯ ½ cup/50 g

CHECK IN

Did you feel satisfied after each meal?

Did you have cravings today?

What's one thing you were grateful for today?

Today's Date:

FOOD AND FITNESS LOG

EXERCISE

LUNCH

BREAKFAST

SNACK

SNACK

DINNER

DAILY NEEDS

WATER		
○ 8 oz/240 ml	○ 8 oz/240 ml	
○ 8 oz/240 ml	○ 8 oz/240 ml	
○ 8 oz/240 ml	○ 8 oz/240 ml	
○ 8 oz/240 ml	○ 8 oz/240 ml	
○ 8 oz/240 ml	○ 8 oz/240 ml	

PROTEIN
○ 4 oz/115 g   ○ 4 oz/115 g
○ 4 oz/115 g   ○ 4 oz/115 g

FAT
○ 1 tbsp   ○ 1 tbsp
○ 1 tbsp

LOW-SUGAR VEGGIES
○ ½ cup/50 g   ○ ½ cup/50 g
○ ½ cup/50 g   ○ ½ cup/50 g
○ ½ cup/50 g   ○ ½ cup/50 g

COMPLEX CARBS
○ ½ cup/50 g   ○ ½ cup/50 g

LOW-SUGAR FRUITS
○ ½ cup/50 g   ○ ½ cup/50 g
○ ½ cup/50 g   ○ ½ cup/50 g

CHECK IN

Did you feel satisfied after each meal?

Did you have cravings today?

What's one thing you were grateful for today?

Today's Date:

FOOD AND FITNESS LOG

EXERCISE

LUNCH

BREAKFAST

SNACK

SNACK

DINNER

DAILY NEEDS

WATER		
	○ 8 oz/240 ml	○ 8 oz/240 ml
	○ 8 oz/240 ml	○ 8 oz/240 ml
	○ 8 oz/240 ml	○ 8 oz/240 ml
	○ 8 oz/240 ml	○ 8 oz/240 ml
	○ 8 oz/240 ml	○ 8 oz/240 ml

PROTEIN		
	○ 4 oz/115 g	○ 4 oz/115 g
	○ 4 oz/115 g	○ 4 oz/115 g

FAT		
	○ 1 tbsp	○ 1 tbsp
	○ 1 tbsp	

LOW-SUGAR VEGGIES		
	○ ½ cup/50 g	○ ½ cup/50 g
	○ ½ cup/50 g	○ ½ cup/50 g
	○ ½ cup/50 g	○ ½ cup/50 g

COMPLEX CARBS		
	○ ½ cup/50 g	○ ½ cup/50 g

LOW-SUGAR FRUITS		
	○ ½ cup/50 g	○ ½ cup/50 g
	○ ½ cup/50 g	○ ½ cup/50 g

CHECK IN

Did you feel satisfied after each meal?

Did you have cravings today?

What's one thing you were grateful for today?

Today's Date:

EXERCISE

LUNCH

_____

BREAKFAST

SNACK

_____

SNACK

DINNER

DAILY NEEDS

WATER
- ◯ 8 oz/240 ml   ◯ 8 oz/240 ml
- ◯ 8 oz/240 ml   ◯ 8 oz/240 ml
- ◯ 8 oz/240 ml   ◯ 8 oz/240 ml
- ◯ 8 oz/240 ml   ◯ 8 oz/240 ml
- ◯ 8 oz/240 ml   ◯ 8 oz/240 ml

PROTEIN
- ◯ 4 oz/115 g   ◯ 4 oz/115 g
- ◯ 4 oz/115 g   ◯ 4 oz/115 g

FAT
- ◯ 1 tbsp   ◯ 1 tbsp
- ◯ 1 tbsp

LOW-SUGAR VEGGIES
- ◯ ½ cup/50 g   ◯ ½ cup/50 g
- ◯ ½ cup/50 g   ◯ ½ cup/50 g
- ◯ ½ cup/50 g   ◯ ½ cup/50 g

COMPLEX CARBS
- ◯ ½ cup/50 g   ◯ ½ cup/50 g

LOW-SUGAR FRUITS
- ◯ ½ cup/50 g   ◯ ½ cup/50 g
- ◯ ½ cup/50 g   ◯ ½ cup/50 g

CHECK IN

Did you feel satisfied after each meal?

_____

Did you have cravings today?

_____

What's one thing you were grateful for today?

_____

Today's Date:

FOOD AND FITNESS LOG

EXERCISE

LUNCH

BREAKFAST

SNACK

SNACK

DINNER

DAILY NEEDS

WATER		
	◯ 8 oz/240 ml	◯ 8 oz/240 ml
	◯ 8 oz/240 ml	◯ 8 oz/240 ml
	◯ 8 oz/240 ml	◯ 8 oz/240 ml
	◯ 8 oz/240 ml	◯ 8 oz/240 ml
	◯ 8 oz/240 ml	◯ 8 oz/240 ml

PROTEIN		
	◯ 4 oz/115 g	◯ 4 oz/115 g
	◯ 4 oz/115 g	◯ 4 oz/115 g

FAT		
	◯ 1 tbsp	◯ 1 tbsp
	◯ 1 tbsp	

LOW-SUGAR VEGGIES		
	◯ ½ cup/50 g	◯ ½ cup/50 g
	◯ ½ cup/50 g	◯ ½ cup/50 g
	◯ ½ cup/50 g	◯ ½ cup/50 g

COMPLEX CARBS		
	◯ ½ cup/50 g	◯ ½ cup/50 g

LOW-SUGAR FRUITS		
	◯ ½ cup/50 g	◯ ½ cup/50 g
	◯ ½ cup/50 g	◯ ½ cup/50 g

CHECK IN

Did you feel satisfied after each meal?

Did you have cravings today?

What's one thing you were grateful for today?

Today's Date:

EXERCISE

LUNCH

BREAKFAST

SNACK

SNACK

DINNER

DAILY NEEDS

WATER		
◯ 8 oz/240 ml	◯ 8 oz/240 ml
◯ 8 oz/240 ml	◯ 8 oz/240 ml
◯ 8 oz/240 ml	◯ 8 oz/240 ml
◯ 8 oz/240 ml	◯ 8 oz/240 ml
◯ 8 oz/240 ml	◯ 8 oz/240 ml

PROTEIN
◯ 4 oz/115 g   ◯ 4 oz/115 g
◯ 4 oz/115 g   ◯ 4 oz/115 g

FAT
◯ 1 tbsp   ◯ 1 tbsp
◯ 1 tbsp

LOW-SUGAR VEGGIES
◯ ½ cup/50 g   ◯ ½ cup/50 g
◯ ½ cup/50 g   ◯ ½ cup/50 g
◯ ½ cup/50 g   ◯ ½ cup/50 g

COMPLEX CARBS
◯ ½ cup/50 g   ◯ ½ cup/50 g

LOW-SUGAR FRUITS
◯ ½ cup/50 g   ◯ ½ cup/50 g
◯ ½ cup/50 g   ◯ ½ cup/50 g

CHECK IN

Did you feel satisfied after each meal?

Did you have cravings today?

What's one thing you were grateful for today?

Today's Date:

EXERCISE

LUNCH

BREAKFAST

SNACK

SNACK

DINNER

SPLURGE

DAILY NEEDS

WATER
- ◯ 8 oz/240 ml
- ◯ 8 oz/240 ml
- ◯ 8 oz/240 ml
- ◯ 8 oz/240 ml
- ◯ 8 oz/240 ml
- ◯ 8 oz/240 ml
- ◯ 8 oz/240 ml
- ◯ 8 oz/240 ml
- ◯ 8 oz/240 ml
- ◯ 8 oz/240 ml

PROTEIN
- ◯ 4 oz/115 g
- ◯ 4 oz/115 g
- ◯ 4 oz/115 g
- ◯ 4 oz/115 g

FAT
- ◯ 1 tbsp
- ◯ 1 tbsp
- ◯ 1 tbsp

LOW-SUGAR VEGGIES
- ◯ ½ cup/50 g
- ◯ ½ cup/50 g
- ◯ ½ cup/50 g
- ◯ ½ cup/50 g
- ◯ ½ cup/50 g
- ◯ ½ cup/50 g

COMPLEX CARBS
- ◯ ½ cup/50 g
- ◯ ½ cup/50 g

LOW-SUGAR FRUITS
- ◯ ½ cup/50 g
- ◯ ½ cup/50 g
- ◯ ½ cup/50 g
- ◯ ½ cup/50 g

CHECK IN

Did you feel satisfied after each meal?

Did you have cravings today?

What's one thing you were grateful for today?

Today's Date:

FOOD AND FITNESS LOG

EXERCISE

LUNCH

BREAKFAST

SNACK

SNACK

DINNER

DAILY NEEDS

WATER

◯ 8 oz/240 ml ◯ 8 oz/240 ml
◯ 8 oz/240 ml ◯ 8 oz/240 ml
◯ 8 oz/240 ml ◯ 8 oz/240 ml
◯ 8 oz/240 ml ◯ 8 oz/240 ml
◯ 8 oz/240 ml ◯ 8 oz/240 ml

PROTEIN

◯ 4 oz/115 g ◯ 4 oz/115 g
◯ 4 oz/115 g ◯ 4 oz/115 g

FAT

◯ 1 tbsp ◯ 1 tbsp
◯ 1 tbsp

LOW-SUGAR VEGGIES

◯ ½ cup/50 g ◯ ½ cup/50 g
◯ ½ cup/50 g ◯ ½ cup/50 g
◯ ½ cup/50 g ◯ ½ cup/50 g

COMPLEX CARBS

◯ ½ cup/50 g ◯ ½ cup/50 g

LOW-SUGAR FRUITS

◯ ½ cup/50 g ◯ ½ cup/50 g
◯ ½ cup/50 g ◯ ½ cup/50 g

CHECK IN

Did you feel satisfied after each meal?

Did you have cravings today?

What's one thing you were grateful for today?

Today's Date:

EXERCISE

LUNCH

BREAKFAST

SNACK

SNACK

DINNER

DAILY NEEDS

WATER		
	◯ 8 oz/240 ml	◯ 8 oz/240 ml
	◯ 8 oz/240 ml	◯ 8 oz/240 ml
	◯ 8 oz/240 ml	◯ 8 oz/240 ml
	◯ 8 oz/240 ml	◯ 8 oz/240 ml
	◯ 8 oz/240 ml	◯ 8 oz/240 ml

PROTEIN		
	◯ 4 oz/115 g	◯ 4 oz/115 g
	◯ 4 oz/115 g	◯ 4 oz/115 g

FAT		
	◯ 1 tbsp	◯ 1 tbsp
	◯ 1 tbsp	

LOW-SUGAR VEGGIES		
	◯ ½ cup/50 g	◯ ½ cup/50 g
	◯ ½ cup/50 g	◯ ½ cup/50 g
	◯ ½ cup/50 g	◯ ½ cup/50 g

COMPLEX CARBS		
	◯ ½ cup/50 g	◯ ½ cup/50 g

LOW-SUGAR FRUITS		
	◯ ½ cup/50 g	◯ ½ cup/50 g
	◯ ½ cup/50 g	◯ ½ cup/50 g

CHECK IN

Did you feel satisfied after each meal?

Did you have cravings today?

What's one thing you were grateful for today?

Today's Date:

FOOD AND FITNESS LOG

EXERCISE

LUNCH

BREAKFAST

SNACK

SNACK

DINNER

DAILY NEEDS

WATER

○ 8 oz/240 ml   ○ 8 oz/240 ml
○ 8 oz/240 ml   ○ 8 oz/240 ml
○ 8 oz/240 ml   ○ 8 oz/240 ml
○ 8 oz/240 ml   ○ 8 oz/240 ml
○ 8 oz/240 ml   ○ 8 oz/240 ml

PROTEIN

○ 4 oz/115 g   ○ 4 oz/115 g
○ 4 oz/115 g   ○ 4 oz/115 g

FAT

○ 1 tbsp   ○ 1 tbsp
○ 1 tbsp

LOW-SUGAR VEGGIES

○ ½ cup/50 g   ○ ½ cup/50 g
○ ½ cup/50 g   ○ ½ cup/50 g
○ ½ cup/50 g   ○ ½ cup/50 g

COMPLEX CARBS

○ ½ cup/50 g   ○ ½ cup/50 g

LOW-SUGAR FRUITS

○ ½ cup/50 g   ○ ½ cup/50 g
○ ½ cup/50 g   ○ ½ cup/50 g

CHECK IN

Did you feel satisfied after each meal?

Did you have cravings today?

What's one thing you were grateful for today?

Today's Date:

FOOD AND FITNESS LOG

EXERCISE

LUNCH

BREAKFAST

SNACK

SNACK

DINNER

DAILY NEEDS

WATER		
◯ 8 oz/240 ml	◯ 8 oz/240 ml	
◯ 8 oz/240 ml	◯ 8 oz/240 ml	
◯ 8 oz/240 ml	◯ 8 oz/240 ml	
◯ 8 oz/240 ml	◯ 8 oz/240 ml	
◯ 8 oz/240 ml	◯ 8 oz/240 ml	

PROTEIN
◯ 4 oz/115 g   ◯ 4 oz/115 g
◯ 4 oz/115 g   ◯ 4 oz/115 g

FAT
◯ 1 tbsp   ◯ 1 tbsp
◯ 1 tbsp

LOW-SUGAR VEGGIES
◯ ½ cup/50 g   ◯ ½ cup/50 g
◯ ½ cup/50 g   ◯ ½ cup/50 g
◯ ½ cup/50 g   ◯ ½ cup/50 g

COMPLEX CARBS
◯ ½ cup/50 g   ◯ ½ cup/50 g

LOW-SUGAR FRUITS
◯ ½ cup/50 g   ◯ ½ cup/50 g
◯ ½ cup/50 g   ◯ ½ cup/50 g

CHECK IN

Did you feel satisfied after each meal?

Did you have cravings today?

What's one thing you were grateful for today?

Today's Date:

EXERCISE

LUNCH

_____

BREAKFAST

SNACK

_____

SNACK

DINNER

DAILY NEEDS

WATER
- ◯ 8 oz/240 ml
- ◯ 8 oz/240 ml
- ◯ 8 oz/240 ml
- ◯ 8 oz/240 ml
- ◯ 8 oz/240 ml

- ◯ 8 oz/240 ml
- ◯ 8 oz/240 ml
- ◯ 8 oz/240 ml
- ◯ 8 oz/240 ml
- ◯ 8 oz/240 ml

LOW-SUGAR VEGGIES
- ◯ ½ cup/50 g
- ◯ ½ cup/50 g
- ◯ ½ cup/50 g

- ◯ ½ cup/50 g
- ◯ ½ cup/50 g
- ◯ ½ cup/50 g

PROTEIN
- ◯ 4 oz/115 g
- ◯ 4 oz/115 g

- ◯ 4 oz/115 g
- ◯ 4 oz/115 g

COMPLEX CARBS
- ◯ ½ cup/50 g

- ◯ ½ cup/50 g

FAT
- ◯ 1 tbsp
- ◯ 1 tbsp

- ◯ 1 tbsp

LOW-SUGAR FRUITS
- ◯ ½ cup/50 g
- ◯ ½ cup/50 g

- ◯ ½ cup/50 g
- ◯ ½ cup/50 g

CHECK IN

Did you feel satisfied after each meal?

_____

Did you have cravings today?

_____

What's one thing you were grateful for today?

_____

Today's Date:

FOOD AND FITNESS LOG

EXERCISE

LUNCH

BREAKFAST

SNACK

SNACK

DINNER

DAILY NEEDS

WATER	◯ 8 oz/240 ml	◯ 8 oz/240 ml
	◯ 8 oz/240 ml	◯ 8 oz/240 ml
	◯ 8 oz/240 ml	◯ 8 oz/240 ml
	◯ 8 oz/240 ml	◯ 8 oz/240 ml
	◯ 8 oz/240 ml	◯ 8 oz/240 ml
PROTEIN	◯ 4 oz/115 g	◯ 4 oz/115 g
	◯ 4 oz/115 g	◯ 4 oz/115 g
FAT	◯ 1 tbsp	◯ 1 tbsp
	◯ 1 tbsp	

LOW-SUGAR VEGGIES	◯ ½ cup/50 g	◯ ½ cup/50 g
	◯ ½ cup/50 g	◯ ½ cup/50 g
	◯ ½ cup/50 g	◯ ½ cup/50 g
COMPLEX CARBS	◯ ½ cup/50 g	◯ ½ cup/50 g
LOW-SUGAR FRUITS	◯ ½ cup/50 g	◯ ½ cup/50 g
	◯ ½ cup/50 g	◯ ½ cup/50 g

CHECK IN

Did you feel satisfied after each meal?

Did you have cravings today?

What's one thing you were grateful for today?

Today's Date:

EXERCISE

LUNCH

BREAKFAST

SNACK

SNACK

DINNER

SPLURGE

DAILY NEEDS

WATER		
◯ 8 oz/240 ml	◯ 8 oz/240 ml	
◯ 8 oz/240 ml	◯ 8 oz/240 ml	
◯ 8 oz/240 ml	◯ 8 oz/240 ml	
◯ 8 oz/240 ml	◯ 8 oz/240 ml	
◯ 8 oz/240 ml	◯ 8 oz/240 ml	

LOW-SUGAR VEGGIES		
◯ ½ cup/50 g	◯ ½ cup/50 g
◯ ½ cup/50 g	◯ ½ cup/50 g
◯ ½ cup/50 g	◯ ½ cup/50 g

COMPLEX CARBS	
◯ ½ cup/50 g	◯ ½ cup/50 g

PROTEIN	
◯ 4 oz/115 g	◯ 4 oz/115 g
◯ 4 oz/115 g	◯ 4 oz/115 g

LOW-SUGAR FRUITS	
◯ ½ cup/50 g	◯ ½ cup/50 g
◯ ½ cup/50 g	◯ ½ cup/50 g

FAT	
◯ 1 tbsp	◯ 1 tbsp
◯ 1 tbsp	

CHECK IN

Did you feel satisfied after each meal?

Did you have cravings today?

What's one thing you were grateful for today?

Today's Date:

FOOD AND FITNESS LOG

EXERCISE

LUNCH

BREAKFAST

SNACK

SNACK

DINNER

DAILY NEEDS

WATER	○ 8 oz/240 ml	○ 8 oz/240 ml	LOW-SUGAR VEGGIES	○ ½ cup/50 g	○ ½ cup/50 g
	○ 8 oz/240 ml	○ 8 oz/240 ml		○ ½ cup/50 g	○ ½ cup/50 g
	○ 8 oz/240 ml	○ 8 oz/240 ml		○ ½ cup/50 g	○ ½ cup/50 g
	○ 8 oz/240 ml	○ 8 oz/240 ml	COMPLEX CARBS	○ ½ cup/50 g	○ ½ cup/50 g
	○ 8 oz/240 ml	○ 8 oz/240 ml			
PROTEIN	○ 4 oz/115 g	○ 4 oz/115 g	LOW-SUGAR FRUITS	○ ½ cup/50 g	○ ½ cup/50 g
	○ 4 oz/115 g	○ 4 oz/115 g		○ ½ cup/50 g	○ ½ cup/50 g
FAT	○ 1 tbsp	○ 1 tbsp			
	○ 1 tbsp				

CHECK IN

Did you feel satisfied after each meal?

Did you have cravings today?

What's one thing you were grateful for today?

Today's Date:

EXERCISE

LUNCH

BREAKFAST

SNACK

SNACK

DINNER

DAILY NEEDS

WATER	◯ 8 oz/240 ml	◯ 8 oz/240 ml
	◯ 8 oz/240 ml	◯ 8 oz/240 ml
	◯ 8 oz/240 ml	◯ 8 oz/240 ml
	◯ 8 oz/240 ml	◯ 8 oz/240 ml
	◯ 8 oz/240 ml	◯ 8 oz/240 ml
PROTEIN	◯ 4 oz/115 g	◯ 4 oz/115 g
	◯ 4 oz/115 g	◯ 4 oz/115 g
FAT	◯ 1 tbsp	◯ 1 tbsp
	◯ 1 tbsp	

LOW-SUGAR VEGGIES	◯ ½ cup/50 g	◯ ½ cup/50 g
	◯ ½ cup/50 g	◯ ½ cup/50 g
	◯ ½ cup/50 g	◯ ½ cup/50 g
COMPLEX CARBS	◯ ½ cup/50 g	◯ ½ cup/50 g
LOW-SUGAR FRUITS	◯ ½ cup/50 g	◯ ½ cup/50 g
	◯ ½ cup/50 g	◯ ½ cup/50 g

CHECK IN

Did you feel satisfied after each meal?

Did you have cravings today?

What's one thing you were grateful for today?

Today's Date:

EXERCISE

LUNCH

BREAKFAST

SNACK

SNACK

DINNER

DAILY NEEDS

WATER

◯ 8 oz/240 ml	◯ 8 oz/240 ml
◯ 8 oz/240 ml	◯ 8 oz/240 ml
◯ 8 oz/240 ml	◯ 8 oz/240 ml
◯ 8 oz/240 ml	◯ 8 oz/240 ml
◯ 8 oz/240 ml	◯ 8 oz/240 ml

PROTEIN

| ◯ 4 oz/115 g | ◯ 4 oz/115 g |
| ◯ 4 oz/115 g | ◯ 4 oz/115 g |

FAT

| ◯ 1 tbsp | ◯ 1 tbsp |
| ◯ 1 tbsp | |

LOW-SUGAR VEGGIES

◯ ½ cup/50 g	◯ ½ cup/50 g
◯ ½ cup/50 g	◯ ½ cup/50 g
◯ ½ cup/50 g	◯ ½ cup/50 g

COMPLEX CARBS

| ◯ ½ cup/50 g | ◯ ½ cup/50 g |

LOW-SUGAR FRUITS

| ◯ ½ cup/50 g | ◯ ½ cup/50 g |
| ◯ ½ cup/50 g | ◯ ½ cup/50 g |

CHECK IN

Did you feel satisfied after each meal?

Did you have cravings today?

What's one thing you were grateful for today?

Today's Date:

EXERCISE

LUNCH

BREAKFAST

SNACK

SNACK

DINNER

DAILY NEEDS

WATER
- 8 oz/240 ml
- 8 oz/240 ml
- 8 oz/240 ml
- 8 oz/240 ml
- 8 oz/240 ml
- 8 oz/240 ml
- 8 oz/240 ml
- 8 oz/240 ml
- 8 oz/240 ml
- 8 oz/240 ml

PROTEIN
- 4 oz/115 g
- 4 oz/115 g
- 4 oz/115 g
- 4 oz/115 g

FAT
- 1 tbsp
- 1 tbsp
- 1 tbsp

LOW-SUGAR VEGGIES
- ½ cup/50 g
- ½ cup/50 g
- ½ cup/50 g
- ½ cup/50 g
- ½ cup/50 g
- ½ cup/50 g

COMPLEX CARBS
- ½ cup/50 g
- ½ cup/50 g

LOW-SUGAR FRUITS
- ½ cup/50 g
- ½ cup/50 g
- ½ cup/50 g
- ½ cup/50 g

CHECK IN

Did you feel satisfied after each meal?

Did you have cravings today?

What's one thing you were grateful for today?

Today's Date:

EXERCISE

LUNCH

BREAKFAST

SNACK

SNACK

DINNER

DAILY NEEDS

WATER	◯ 8 oz/240 ml	◯ 8 oz/240 ml
	◯ 8 oz/240 ml	◯ 8 oz/240 ml
	◯ 8 oz/240 ml	◯ 8 oz/240 ml
	◯ 8 oz/240 ml	◯ 8 oz/240 ml
	◯ 8 oz/240 ml	◯ 8 oz/240 ml
PROTEIN	◯ 4 oz/115 g	◯ 4 oz/115 g
	◯ 4 oz/115 g	◯ 4 oz/115 g
FAT	◯ 1 tbsp	◯ 1 tbsp
	◯ 1 tbsp	

LOW-SUGAR VEGGIES	◯ ½ cup/50 g	◯ ½ cup/50 g
	◯ ½ cup/50 g	◯ ½ cup/50 g
	◯ ½ cup/50 g	◯ ½ cup/50 g
COMPLEX CARBS	◯ ½ cup/50 g	◯ ½ cup/50 g
LOW-SUGAR FRUITS	◯ ½ cup/50 g	◯ ½ cup/50 g
	◯ ½ cup/50 g	◯ ½ cup/50 g

CHECK IN

Did you feel satisfied after each meal?

Did you have cravings today?

What's one thing you were grateful for today?

Today's Date:

EXERCISE

LUNCH

_____

BREAKFAST

SNACK

_____

SNACK

DINNER

DAILY NEEDS

WATER		
◯ 8 oz/240 ml	◯ 8 oz/240 ml
◯ 8 oz/240 ml	◯ 8 oz/240 ml
◯ 8 oz/240 ml	◯ 8 oz/240 ml
◯ 8 oz/240 ml	◯ 8 oz/240 ml
◯ 8 oz/240 ml	◯ 8 oz/240 ml

PROTEIN
◯ 4 oz/115 g   ◯ 4 oz/115 g
◯ 4 oz/115 g   ◯ 4 oz/115 g

FAT
◯ 1 tbsp   ◯ 1 tbsp
◯ 1 tbsp

LOW-SUGAR VEGGIES
◯ ½ cup/50 g   ◯ ½ cup/50 g
◯ ½ cup/50 g   ◯ ½ cup/50 g
◯ ½ cup/50 g   ◯ ½ cup/50 g

COMPLEX CARBS
◯ ½ cup/50 g   ◯ ½ cup/50 g

LOW-SUGAR FRUITS
◯ ½ cup/50 g   ◯ ½ cup/50 g
◯ ½ cup/50 g   ◯ ½ cup/50 g

CHECK IN

Did you feel satisfied after each meal?

_____

Did you have cravings today?

_____

What's one thing you were grateful for today?

_____

Today's Date:

EXERCISE

LUNCH

BREAKFAST

SNACK

SNACK

DINNER

SPLURGE

DAILY NEEDS

WATER		
◯ 8 oz/240 ml	◯ 8 oz/240 ml	
◯ 8 oz/240 ml	◯ 8 oz/240 ml	
◯ 8 oz/240 ml	◯ 8 oz/240 ml	
◯ 8 oz/240 ml	◯ 8 oz/240 ml	
◯ 8 oz/240 ml	◯ 8 oz/240 ml	

PROTEIN	
◯ 4 oz/115 g	◯ 4 oz/115 g
◯ 4 oz/115 g	◯ 4 oz/115 g

FAT	
◯ 1 tbsp	◯ 1 tbsp
◯ 1 tbsp	

LOW-SUGAR VEGGIES	
◯ ½ cup/50 g	◯ ½ cup/50 g
◯ ½ cup/50 g	◯ ½ cup/50 g
◯ ½ cup/50 g	◯ ½ cup/50 g

COMPLEX CARBS	
◯ ½ cup/50 g	◯ ½ cup/50 g

LOW-SUGAR FRUITS	
◯ ½ cup/50 g	◯ ½ cup/50 g
◯ ½ cup/50 g	◯ ½ cup/50 g

CHECK IN

Did you feel satisfied after each meal?

Did you have cravings today?

What's one thing you were grateful for today?

Today's Date:

FOOD AND FITNESS LOG

EXERCISE

LUNCH

BREAKFAST

SNACK

SNACK

DINNER

DAILY NEEDS

WATER	◯ 8 oz/240 ml	◯ 8 oz/240 ml
	◯ 8 oz/240 ml	◯ 8 oz/240 ml
	◯ 8 oz/240 ml	◯ 8 oz/240 ml
	◯ 8 oz/240 ml	◯ 8 oz/240 ml
	◯ 8 oz/240 ml	◯ 8 oz/240 ml
PROTEIN	◯ 4 oz/115 g	◯ 4 oz/115 g
	◯ 4 oz/115 g	◯ 4 oz/115 g
FAT	◯ 1 tbsp	◯ 1 tbsp
	◯ 1 tbsp	

LOW-SUGAR VEGGIES	◯ ½ cup/50 g	◯ ½ cup/50 g
	◯ ½ cup/50 g	◯ ½ cup/50 g
	◯ ½ cup/50 g	◯ ½ cup/50 g
COMPLEX CARBS	◯ ½ cup/50 g	◯ ½ cup/50 g
LOW-SUGAR FRUITS	◯ ½ cup/50 g	◯ ½ cup/50 g
	◯ ½ cup/50 g	◯ ½ cup/50 g

CHECK IN

Did you feel satisfied after each meal?

Did you have cravings today?

What's one thing you were grateful for today?

Today's Date:

EXERCISE

LUNCH

BREAKFAST

SNACK

SNACK

DINNER

DAILY NEEDS

WATER

○ 8 oz/240 ml   ○ 8 oz/240 ml
○ 8 oz/240 ml   ○ 8 oz/240 ml
○ 8 oz/240 ml   ○ 8 oz/240 ml
○ 8 oz/240 ml   ○ 8 oz/240 ml
○ 8 oz/240 ml   ○ 8 oz/240 ml

PROTEIN

○ 4 oz/115 g   ○ 4 oz/115 g
○ 4 oz/115 g   ○ 4 oz/115 g

FAT

○ 1 tbsp   ○ 1 tbsp
○ 1 tbsp

LOW-SUGAR VEGGIES

○ ½ cup/50 g   ○ ½ cup/50 g
○ ½ cup/50 g   ○ ½ cup/50 g
○ ½ cup/50 g   ○ ½ cup/50 g

COMPLEX CARBS

○ ½ cup/50 g   ○ ½ cup/50 g

LOW-SUGAR FRUITS

○ ½ cup/50 g   ○ ½ cup/50 g
○ ½ cup/50 g   ○ ½ cup/50 g

CHECK IN

Did you feel satisfied after each meal?

Did you have cravings today?

What's one thing you were grateful for today?

Today's Date:

EXERCISE

LUNCH

BREAKFAST

SNACK

SNACK

DINNER

DAILY NEEDS

WATER
- ( ) 8 oz/240 ml
- ( ) 8 oz/240 ml
- ( ) 8 oz/240 ml
- ( ) 8 oz/240 ml
- ( ) 8 oz/240 ml

- ( ) 8 oz/240 ml
- ( ) 8 oz/240 ml
- ( ) 8 oz/240 ml
- ( ) 8 oz/240 ml
- ( ) 8 oz/240 ml

PROTEIN
- ( ) 4 oz/115 g
- ( ) 4 oz/115 g

- ( ) 4 oz/115 g
- ( ) 4 oz/115 g

FAT
- ( ) 1 tbsp
- ( ) 1 tbsp

- ( ) 1 tbsp

LOW-SUGAR VEGGIES
- ( ) ½ cup/50 g
- ( ) ½ cup/50 g
- ( ) ½ cup/50 g

- ( ) ½ cup/50 g
- ( ) ½ cup/50 g
- ( ) ½ cup/50 g

COMPLEX CARBS
- ( ) ½ cup/50 g

- ( ) ½ cup/50 g

LOW-SUGAR FRUITS
- ( ) ½ cup/50 g
- ( ) ½ cup/50 g

- ( ) ½ cup/50 g
- ( ) ½ cup/50 g

CHECK IN

Did you feel satisfied after each meal?

Did you have cravings today?

What's one thing you were grateful for today?

Today's Date:

FOOD AND FITNESS LOG

EXERCISE

LUNCH

BREAKFAST

SNACK

SNACK

DINNER

DAILY NEEDS

WATER
- ◯ 8 oz/240 ml
- ◯ 8 oz/240 ml
- ◯ 8 oz/240 ml
- ◯ 8 oz/240 ml
- ◯ 8 oz/240 ml

- ◯ 8 oz/240 ml
- ◯ 8 oz/240 ml
- ◯ 8 oz/240 ml
- ◯ 8 oz/240 ml
- ◯ 8 oz/240 ml

PROTEIN
- ◯ 4 oz/115 g
- ◯ 4 oz/115 g

- ◯ 4 oz/115 g
- ◯ 4 oz/115 g

FAT
- ◯ 1 tbsp
- ◯ 1 tbsp

- ◯ 1 tbsp

LOW-SUGAR VEGGIES
- ◯ ½ cup/50 g
- ◯ ½ cup/50 g
- ◯ ½ cup/50 g

- ◯ ½ cup/50 g
- ◯ ½ cup/50 g
- ◯ ½ cup/50 g

COMPLEX CARBS
- ◯ ½ cup/50 g

- ◯ ½ cup/50 g

LOW-SUGAR FRUITS
- ◯ ½ cup/50 g
- ◯ ½ cup/50 g

- ◯ ½ cup/50 g
- ◯ ½ cup/50 g

CHECK IN

Did you feel satisfied after each meal?

Did you have cravings today?

What's one thing you were grateful for today?

Today's Date:

EXERCISE

LUNCH

_____

BREAKFAST

SNACK

_____

SNACK

DINNER

DAILY NEEDS

WATER	
○ 8 oz/240 ml	○ 8 oz/240 ml
○ 8 oz/240 ml	○ 8 oz/240 ml
○ 8 oz/240 ml	○ 8 oz/240 ml
○ 8 oz/240 ml	○ 8 oz/240 ml
○ 8 oz/240 ml	○ 8 oz/240 ml

PROTEIN	
○ 4 oz/115 g	○ 4 oz/115 g
○ 4 oz/115 g	○ 4 oz/115 g

FAT	
○ 1 tbsp	○ 1 tbsp
○ 1 tbsp	

LOW-SUGAR VEGGIES	
○ ½ cup/50 g	○ ½ cup/50 g
○ ½ cup/50 g	○ ½ cup/50 g
○ ½ cup/50 g	○ ½ cup/50 g

COMPLEX CARBS	
○ ½ cup/50 g	○ ½ cup/50 g

LOW-SUGAR FRUITS	
○ ½ cup/50 g	○ ½ cup/50 g
○ ½ cup/50 g	○ ½ cup/50 g

CHECK IN

Did you feel satisfied after each meal?

_____

Did you have cravings today?

_____

What's one thing you were grateful for today?

_____

Today's Date:

EXERCISE

LUNCH

BREAKFAST

SNACK

SNACK

DINNER

DAILY NEEDS

WATER		
○ 8 oz/240 ml	○ 8 oz/240 ml	
○ 8 oz/240 ml	○ 8 oz/240 ml	
○ 8 oz/240 ml	○ 8 oz/240 ml	
○ 8 oz/240 ml	○ 8 oz/240 ml	
○ 8 oz/240 ml	○ 8 oz/240 ml	

PROTEIN	
○ 4 oz/115 g	○ 4 oz/115 g
○ 4 oz/115 g	○ 4 oz/115 g

FAT	
○ 1 tbsp	○ 1 tbsp
○ 1 tbsp	

LOW-SUGAR VEGGIES
○ ½ cup/50 g   ○ ½ cup/50 g
○ ½ cup/50 g   ○ ½ cup/50 g
○ ½ cup/50 g   ○ ½ cup/50 g

COMPLEX CARBS
○ ½ cup/50 g   ○ ½ cup/50 g

LOW-SUGAR FRUITS
○ ½ cup/50 g   ○ ½ cup/50 g
○ ½ cup/50 g   ○ ½ cup/50 g

CHECK IN

Did you feel satisfied after each meal?

Did you have cravings today?

What's one thing you were grateful for today?

Today's Date:

EXERCISE

LUNCH

BREAKFAST

SNACK

SNACK

DINNER

SPLURGE

DAILY NEEDS

WATER		
	○ 8 oz/240 ml	○ 8 oz/240 ml
	○ 8 oz/240 ml	○ 8 oz/240 ml
	○ 8 oz/240 ml	○ 8 oz/240 ml
	○ 8 oz/240 ml	○ 8 oz/240 ml
	○ 8 oz/240 ml	○ 8 oz/240 ml

PROTEIN
○ 4 oz/115 g   ○ 4 oz/115 g
○ 4 oz/115 g   ○ 4 oz/115 g

FAT
○ 1 tbsp   ○ 1 tbsp
○ 1 tbsp

LOW-SUGAR VEGGIES
○ ½ cup/50 g   ○ ½ cup/50 g
○ ½ cup/50 g   ○ ½ cup/50 g
○ ½ cup/50 g   ○ ½ cup/50 g

COMPLEX CARBS
○ ½ cup/50 g   ○ ½ cup/50 g

LOW-SUGAR FRUITS
○ ½ cup/50 g   ○ ½ cup/50 g
○ ½ cup/50 g   ○ ½ cup/50 g

CHECK IN

Did you feel satisfied after each meal?

Did you have cravings today?

What's one thing you were grateful for today?

Today's Date:

EXERCISE

LUNCH

BREAKFAST

SNACK

SNACK

DINNER

DAILY NEEDS

WATER
- ◯ 8 oz/240 ml
- ◯ 8 oz/240 ml
- ◯ 8 oz/240 ml
- ◯ 8 oz/240 ml
- ◯ 8 oz/240 ml

- ◯ 8 oz/240 ml
- ◯ 8 oz/240 ml
- ◯ 8 oz/240 ml
- ◯ 8 oz/240 ml
- ◯ 8 oz/240 ml

PROTEIN
- ◯ 4 oz/115 g
- ◯ 4 oz/115 g

- ◯ 4 oz/115 g
- ◯ 4 oz/115 g

FAT
- ◯ 1 tbsp
- ◯ 1 tbsp

- ◯ 1 tbsp

LOW-SUGAR VEGGIES
- ◯ ½ cup/50 g
- ◯ ½ cup/50 g
- ◯ ½ cup/50 g

- ◯ ½ cup/50 g
- ◯ ½ cup/50 g
- ◯ ½ cup/50 g

COMPLEX CARBS
- ◯ ½ cup/50 g

- ◯ ½ cup/50 g

LOW-SUGAR FRUITS
- ◯ ½ cup/50 g
- ◯ ½ cup/50 g

- ◯ ½ cup/50 g
- ◯ ½ cup/50 g

CHECK IN

Did you feel satisfied after each meal?

Did you have cravings today?

What's one thing you were grateful for today?

Today's Date:

EXERCISE

LUNCH

BREAKFAST

SNACK

SNACK

DINNER

DAILY NEEDS

WATER		
	○ 8 oz/240 ml	○ 8 oz/240 ml
	○ 8 oz/240 ml	○ 8 oz/240 ml
	○ 8 oz/240 ml	○ 8 oz/240 ml
	○ 8 oz/240 ml	○ 8 oz/240 ml
	○ 8 oz/240 ml	○ 8 oz/240 ml

PROTEIN		
	○ 4 oz/115 g	○ 4 oz/115 g
	○ 4 oz/115 g	○ 4 oz/115 g

FAT		
	○ 1 tbsp	○ 1 tbsp
	○ 1 tbsp	

LOW-SUGAR VEGGIES		
	○ ½ cup/50 g	○ ½ cup/50 g
	○ ½ cup/50 g	○ ½ cup/50 g
	○ ½ cup/50 g	○ ½ cup/50 g

COMPLEX CARBS		
	○ ½ cup/50 g	○ ½ cup/50 g

LOW-SUGAR FRUITS		
	○ ½ cup/50 g	○ ½ cup/50 g
	○ ½ cup/50 g	○ ½ cup/50 g

CHECK IN

Did you feel satisfied after each meal?

Did you have cravings today?

What's one thing you were grateful for today?

Today's Date:

FOOD AND FITNESS LOG

EXERCISE

LUNCH

BREAKFAST

SNACK

SNACK

DINNER

DAILY NEEDS

WATER

- ◯ 8 oz/240 ml
- ◯ 8 oz/240 ml
- ◯ 8 oz/240 ml
- ◯ 8 oz/240 ml
- ◯ 8 oz/240 ml

- ◯ 8 oz/240 ml
- ◯ 8 oz/240 ml
- ◯ 8 oz/240 ml
- ◯ 8 oz/240 ml
- ◯ 8 oz/240 ml

PROTEIN

- ◯ 4 oz/115 g
- ◯ 4 oz/115 g

- ◯ 4 oz/115 g
- ◯ 4 oz/115 g

FAT

- ◯ 1 tbsp
- ◯ 1 tbsp

- ◯ 1 tbsp

LOW-SUGAR VEGGIES

- ◯ ½ cup/50 g
- ◯ ½ cup/50 g
- ◯ ½ cup/50 g

- ◯ ½ cup/50 g
- ◯ ½ cup/50 g
- ◯ ½ cup/50 g

COMPLEX CARBS

- ◯ ½ cup/50 g

- ◯ ½ cup/50 g

LOW-SUGAR FRUITS

- ◯ ½ cup/50 g
- ◯ ½ cup/50 g

- ◯ ½ cup/50 g
- ◯ ½ cup/50 g

CHECK IN

Did you feel satisfied after each meal?

Did you have cravings today?

What's one thing you were grateful for today?

Today's Date:

EXERCISE

LUNCH

BREAKFAST

SNACK

SNACK

DINNER

DAILY NEEDS

WATER
- ◯ 8 oz/240 ml
- ◯ 8 oz/240 ml
- ◯ 8 oz/240 ml
- ◯ 8 oz/240 ml
- ◯ 8 oz/240 ml

- ◯ 8 oz/240 ml
- ◯ 8 oz/240 ml
- ◯ 8 oz/240 ml
- ◯ 8 oz/240 ml
- ◯ 8 oz/240 ml

PROTEIN
- ◯ 4 oz/115 g
- ◯ 4 oz/115 g

- ◯ 4 oz/115 g
- ◯ 4 oz/115 g

FAT
- ◯ 1 tbsp
- ◯ 1 tbsp

- ◯ 1 tbsp

LOW-SUGAR VEGGIES
- ◯ ½ cup/50 g
- ◯ ½ cup/50 g
- ◯ ½ cup/50 g

- ◯ ½ cup/50 g
- ◯ ½ cup/50 g
- ◯ ½ cup/50 g

COMPLEX CARBS
- ◯ ½ cup/50 g

- ◯ ½ cup/50 g

LOW-SUGAR FRUITS
- ◯ ½ cup/50 g
- ◯ ½ cup/50 g

- ◯ ½ cup/50 g
- ◯ ½ cup/50 g

CHECK IN

Did you feel satisfied after each meal?

Did you have cravings today?

What's one thing you were grateful for today?

Today's Date:

FOOD AND FITNESS LOG

EXERCISE

LUNCH

BREAKFAST

SNACK

SNACK

DINNER

DAILY NEEDS

WATER
- ◯ 8 oz/240 ml
- ◯ 8 oz/240 ml
- ◯ 8 oz/240 ml
- ◯ 8 oz/240 ml
- ◯ 8 oz/240 ml
- ◯ 8 oz/240 ml
- ◯ 8 oz/240 ml
- ◯ 8 oz/240 ml
- ◯ 8 oz/240 ml
- ◯ 8 oz/240 ml

PROTEIN
- ◯ 4 oz/115 g
- ◯ 4 oz/115 g
- ◯ 4 oz/115 g
- ◯ 4 oz/115 g

FAT
- ◯ 1 tbsp
- ◯ 1 tbsp
- ◯ 1 tbsp

LOW-SUGAR VEGGIES
- ◯ ½ cup/50 g
- ◯ ½ cup/50 g
- ◯ ½ cup/50 g
- ◯ ½ cup/50 g
- ◯ ½ cup/50 g
- ◯ ½ cup/50 g

COMPLEX CARBS
- ◯ ½ cup/50 g
- ◯ ½ cup/50 g

LOW-SUGAR FRUITS
- ◯ ½ cup/50 g
- ◯ ½ cup/50 g
- ◯ ½ cup/50 g
- ◯ ½ cup/50 g

CHECK IN

Did you feel satisfied after each meal?

Did you have cravings today?

What's one thing you were grateful for today?

Today's Date:

EXERCISE

LUNCH

BREAKFAST

SNACK

SNACK

DINNER

DAILY NEEDS

WATER
- ◯ 8 oz/240 ml   ◯ 8 oz/240 ml
- ◯ 8 oz/240 ml   ◯ 8 oz/240 ml
- ◯ 8 oz/240 ml   ◯ 8 oz/240 ml
- ◯ 8 oz/240 ml   ◯ 8 oz/240 ml
- ◯ 8 oz/240 ml   ◯ 8 oz/240 ml

PROTEIN
- ◯ 4 oz/115 g   ◯ 4 oz/115 g
- ◯ 4 oz/115 g   ◯ 4 oz/115 g

FAT
- ◯ 1 tbsp   ◯ 1 tbsp
- ◯ 1 tbsp

LOW-SUGAR VEGGIES
- ◯ ½ cup/50 g   ◯ ½ cup/50 g
- ◯ ½ cup/50 g   ◯ ½ cup/50 g
- ◯ ½ cup/50 g   ◯ ½ cup/50 g

COMPLEX CARBS
- ◯ ½ cup/50 g   ◯ ½ cup/50 g

LOW-SUGAR FRUITS
- ◯ ½ cup/50 g   ◯ ½ cup/50 g
- ◯ ½ cup/50 g   ◯ ½ cup/50 g

CHECK IN

Did you feel satisfied after each meal?

Did you have cravings today?

What's one thing you were grateful for today?

Today's Date:

EXERCISE

LUNCH

_____

BREAKFAST

SNACK

_____

SNACK

DINNER

_____

SPLURGE

DAILY NEEDS

WATER		
◯ 8 oz/240 ml	◯ 8 oz/240 ml
◯ 8 oz/240 ml	◯ 8 oz/240 ml
◯ 8 oz/240 ml	◯ 8 oz/240 ml
◯ 8 oz/240 ml	◯ 8 oz/240 ml
◯ 8 oz/240 ml	◯ 8 oz/240 ml

LOW-SUGAR VEGGIES
◯ ½ cup/50 g   ◯ ½ cup/50 g
◯ ½ cup/50 g   ◯ ½ cup/50 g
◯ ½ cup/50 g   ◯ ½ cup/50 g

PROTEIN
◯ 4 oz/115 g   ◯ 4 oz/115 g
◯ 4 oz/115 g   ◯ 4 oz/115 g

COMPLEX CARBS
◯ ½ cup/50 g   ◯ ½ cup/50 g

FAT
◯ 1 tbsp   ◯ 1 tbsp
◯ 1 tbsp

LOW-SUGAR FRUITS
◯ ½ cup/50 g   ◯ ½ cup/50 g
◯ ½ cup/50 g   ◯ ½ cup/50 g

CHECK IN

Did you feel satisfied after each meal?

_____

Did you have cravings today?

_____

What's one thing you were grateful for today?

_____

Today's Date:

EXERCISE

LUNCH

BREAKFAST

SNACK

SNACK

DINNER

DAILY NEEDS

WATER		
○ 8 oz/240 ml	○ 8 oz/240 ml
○ 8 oz/240 ml	○ 8 oz/240 ml
○ 8 oz/240 ml	○ 8 oz/240 ml
○ 8 oz/240 ml	○ 8 oz/240 ml
○ 8 oz/240 ml	○ 8 oz/240 ml

PROTEIN	
○ 4 oz/115 g	○ 4 oz/115 g
○ 4 oz/115 g	○ 4 oz/115 g

FAT	
○ 1 tbsp	○ 1 tbsp
○ 1 tbsp	

LOW-SUGAR VEGGIES
○ ½ cup/50 g   ○ ½ cup/50 g
○ ½ cup/50 g   ○ ½ cup/50 g
○ ½ cup/50 g   ○ ½ cup/50 g

COMPLEX CARBS
○ ½ cup/50 g   ○ ½ cup/50 g

LOW-SUGAR FRUITS
○ ½ cup/50 g   ○ ½ cup/50 g
○ ½ cup/50 g   ○ ½ cup/50 g

CHECK IN

Did you feel satisfied after each meal?

Did you have cravings today?

What's one thing you were grateful for today?

Today's Date:

FOOD AND FITNESS LOG

EXERCISE

LUNCH

BREAKFAST

SNACK

SNACK

DINNER

DAILY NEEDS

WATER
- ◯ 8 oz/240 ml
- ◯ 8 oz/240 ml
- ◯ 8 oz/240 ml
- ◯ 8 oz/240 ml
- ◯ 8 oz/240 ml
- ◯ 8 oz/240 ml
- ◯ 8 oz/240 ml
- ◯ 8 oz/240 ml
- ◯ 8 oz/240 ml
- ◯ 8 oz/240 ml

PROTEIN
- ◯ 4 oz/115 g
- ◯ 4 oz/115 g
- ◯ 4 oz/115 g
- ◯ 4 oz/115 g

FAT
- ◯ 1 tbsp
- ◯ 1 tbsp
- ◯ 1 tbsp

LOW-SUGAR VEGGIES
- ◯ ½ cup/50 g
- ◯ ½ cup/50 g
- ◯ ½ cup/50 g
- ◯ ½ cup/50 g
- ◯ ½ cup/50 g
- ◯ ½ cup/50 g

COMPLEX CARBS
- ◯ ½ cup/50 g
- ◯ ½ cup/50 g

LOW-SUGAR FRUITS
- ◯ ½ cup/50 g
- ◯ ½ cup/50 g
- ◯ ½ cup/50 g
- ◯ ½ cup/50 g

CHECK IN

Did you feel satisfied after each meal?

Did you have cravings today?

What's one thing you were grateful for today?

Today's Date:

FOOD AND FITNESS LOG

EXERCISE

LUNCH

BREAKFAST

SNACK

SNACK

DINNER

DAILY NEEDS

WATER	◯ 8 oz/240 ml	◯ 8 oz/240 ml
	◯ 8 oz/240 ml	◯ 8 oz/240 ml
	◯ 8 oz/240 ml	◯ 8 oz/240 ml
	◯ 8 oz/240 ml	◯ 8 oz/240 ml
	◯ 8 oz/240 ml	◯ 8 oz/240 ml
PROTEIN	◯ 4 oz/115 g	◯ 4 oz/115 g
	◯ 4 oz/115 g	◯ 4 oz/115 g
FAT	◯ 1 tbsp	◯ 1 tbsp
	◯ 1 tbsp	

LOW-SUGAR VEGGIES	◯ ½ cup/50 g	◯ ½ cup/50 g
	◯ ½ cup/50 g	◯ ½ cup/50 g
	◯ ½ cup/50 g	◯ ½ cup/50 g
COMPLEX CARBS	◯ ½ cup/50 g	◯ ½ cup/50 g
LOW-SUGAR FRUITS	◯ ½ cup/50 g	◯ ½ cup/50 g
	◯ ½ cup/50 g	◯ ½ cup/50 g

CHECK IN

Did you feel satisfied after each meal?

Did you have cravings today?

What's one thing you were grateful for today?

Today's Date:

EXERCISE

LUNCH

BREAKFAST

SNACK

SNACK

DINNER

DAILY NEEDS

WATER				
○ 8 oz/240 ml	○ 8 oz/240 ml			
○ 8 oz/240 ml	○ 8 oz/240 ml			
○ 8 oz/240 ml	○ 8 oz/240 ml			
○ 8 oz/240 ml	○ 8 oz/240 ml			
○ 8 oz/240 ml	○ 8 oz/240 ml			

LOW-SUGAR VEGGIES
○ ½ cup/50 g   ○ ½ cup/50 g
○ ½ cup/50 g   ○ ½ cup/50 g
○ ½ cup/50 g   ○ ½ cup/50 g

COMPLEX CARBS
○ ½ cup/50 g   ○ ½ cup/50 g

PROTEIN
○ 4 oz/115 g   ○ 4 oz/115 g
○ 4 oz/115 g   ○ 4 oz/115 g

LOW-SUGAR FRUITS
○ ½ cup/50 g   ○ ½ cup/50 g
○ ½ cup/50 g   ○ ½ cup/50 g

FAT
○ 1 tbsp   ○ 1 tbsp
○ 1 tbsp

CHECK IN

Did you feel satisfied after each meal?

Did you have cravings today?

What's one thing you were grateful for today?

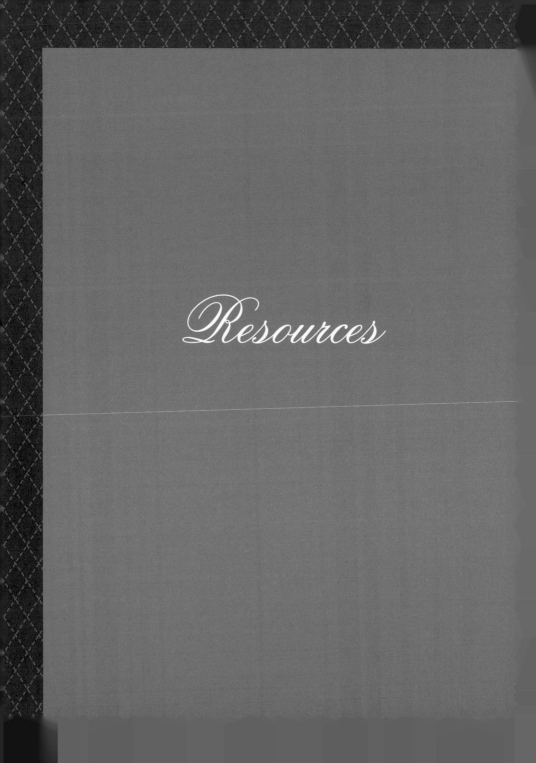

Resources

Web Sites

Biogenesis Protein Bars
www.bio-genesis.com
Gluten- and dairy-free protein bars

Charles Poliquin
www.charlespoliquin.com
*Ball-busting fitness articles,
supplements, and blogs*

Environmental Working Group
www.ewg.org
An environmental awareness resource

Fat-Loss Lifestyle
www.metaboliceffect.com
*Personally tailored workouts and
articles. Also check out* The New ME
Diet *book on the site.*

JillFit Exercise
www.jillfit.com
Customized workouts, articles, and blog

Lumie Light
www.lumie.com
Light-therapy treatments for mind and body

Meditation CDs
www.healthjourneys.com
Belleruth Neparstek's meditations are divine

Non-GMO Foods
www.seedsofdeception.com
www.responsibletechnology.org
*Politics behind GMOs and their
consequences*

Shirataki Noodles
www.shiratakinoodles.net
Gluten-free noodles

Soy Truths
www.thewholesoystory.com
Research studies on the evolution of soy

Supplements
www.designsforhealth.com
Clinical research and supplements

Vitamin D
www.vitamindcouncil.org
*Articles on cutting-edge vitamin D
research*

Wild Alaskan Salmon
www.vitalchoice.com
A sustainable seafood source

Cookbooks

Barefoot Contessa by Ina Garten
Simple, easy recipes anyone can follow

Everyday Paleo by Sarah Fragoso
An amazing resource for paleo-style recipes

The Family Kitchen by Debra Ponzek
Gets your whole family involved in cooking

Harvest to Heat by Darryl Estrine and Kelly Kochendorfer
A great read on sustainable eating

Inspired by Ingredients by Bill Telepan
A chef's cookbook of market-based cooking

Nourishing Traditions by Sally Fallon
Features the importance of traditional foods

Acknowledgments

Special thanks to Team Gorgeous: Kate Woodrow and Celeste Fine. I love our collaborative efforts and the pink bibles we've made together! You both continually inspire me to reach high and stand proud—thank you. I'd also like to thank my friends and colleagues who graciously share their knowledge with me and make my practice richer: Jade Teta and the Metabolic Effect team, Jill Coleman, and Charles Poliquin. Without you, this book would not have been possible.

Thanks to the incredibly talented Brian Delaney for the gorgeous headshots and an amazing day! And thanks to all the peeps who submitted questions for the book, too—you know who you are—and to Nicole Paul for her slop recipe. Last, I'd like to thank my guys at home: Jeremy and Benjamin. I love you to infinity and beyond.

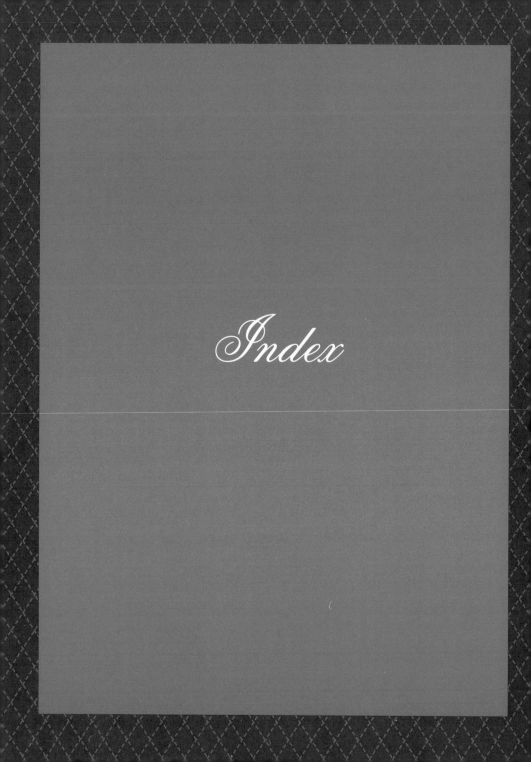

Index